Telling my wife's story of natural home birth that

resulted in a life-changing

C-section.

A simple guide for New Moms on pregnancy care and

childbirth preparations.

Georgandez Morrison

Disclaimer

I'm not a doctor, nutritionist, or a medical professional of any kind. This book is not intended or licensed to treat, diagnose, or heal any pregnancy-related issue. I wrote this book after conducting thorough research, based on the opinions of medical professionals and my wife's pregnancy and childbirth experience. This book is only intended to help you make informed decisions about your health. It's not intended to replace the knowledge and expertise of your health-care provider. Before you include or avoid any of the foods, techniques, or methods mentioned in this book, please consult your health-care provider. Before starting or stopping any treatment or acting upon any information in this book, you should contact your health-care provider.

Acknowledgments

My wife, Tianka Morrison: I admire and will forever remember your relentless strength and courage to birth our child despite the horrendous odds that were against you. Thank you for making me a father. I Love You!

My daughter, Geor'nyah Morrison: Your ability to maintain a steady heartbeat throughout the various methods of delivery is an accurate representation of your inner strength. It's the kind of strength that you will express for the world to see. Thank you for remaining alive! Pa loves you!

Our birth support Team: *To Michelle Williams, Shannon Williams, Keverne Mason, and everyone else who was a part of our birth support team. I am grateful for your selfless toil and assistance in getting our baby girl here safely.*

Our church family: Special thanks to Pastor. Cornelius and Heather Lindsey, Agatha Marshall, and Nadra Cohens. Your support throughout this journey will be forever appreciated and remembered.

why I wrote this book?

Strengthening the foundation of your knowledge about pregnancy and childbirth is one of the best investments you can give to your child and your body. I wrote this book for the moms who are interested in being educated on their health and well-being during pregnancy and childbirth. This book is also written to empower women who want to take control of their pregnancy and childbirth experience from an educational standpoint. My vision for this book is to not throw a bunch of scientific pregnancy-related terminologies and solutions at you and your precious baby. Instead, I want you - the mom, to have an insight of both worlds by simplifying the scientific pregnancy-related terminologies and solutions and also providing a raw, unedited, glimpse of the highs and lows of a real-life pregnancy and childbirth. By sharing my wife's experiences – her highs and lowest moments; I hope that you'll learn lessons that are more valuable than scientific pregnancy-related terminologies and solutions.

Contents

Our Story

Chapter One

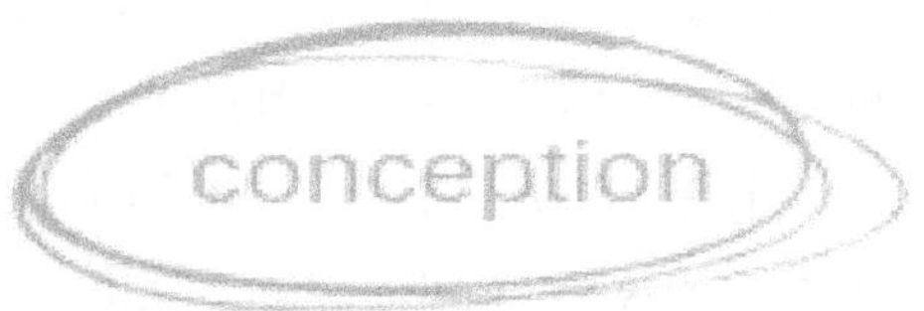

**" *Every beautiful & meaningful journey*
*begins with conception.***

The beautiful innocence in my daughter's eyes always prompts me to reflect on how much my wife and I labored in prayer for a child. The duration of how long we prayed to see life within her eyes wasn't a reflection of how long it took for her to fully develop within the womb. It required three additional months on top of the forty-one (41) weeks and six (6) days that we waited anxiously for her.

After relentless efforts of trying to conceive for over a year, Tianka finally conceived our first child, Geor'nyah Eliana

Morrison, which means "God's Gift to Us." Her conception was a true depiction of God's perfect timing, favor, and promise in our union. We were both elated!

Before she surprised me with the wonderful news, I had many reasons to suspect that she was already pregnant. Her frequent trips to the bathroom, the subliminal messages that hinted at her being pregnant, my constant dreams of having a baby girl, and my strong urge for fatherhood were enough to ignite a light bulb. However, at the time of my suspicion, I had no solid evidence. Therefore, I tucked the suspicion far away in my mind.

One day after arriving home, she called me inside our bedroom and told me that she had a surprise for me. I began to wonder what this surprise was. We sat on the floor and suddenly, she gave me a children's book. I paused for a second, and without zooming in on the book, the man inside my head began saying, "A book!" I paused for another moment, and I glanced at the title of the book. It was entitled –'You Are My Sunshine,' written by Caroline Jayne Church. Now, at this point, I know you, the readers must be thinking, "He figured it out." Well, unfortunately, like most guys, I still had that clueless look on my face. Muscles knitted across my eyebrows. I asked, "Why are you giving me this?" She chuckled! For a second, I thought she was being a weirdo. I asked myself, "What kind of woman gives an adult male a children's book?" Haha. Little did I know what was about to unfold. She took from underneath our bed another book – 'The Fatherhood Principles' written by the late Dr. Myles Munroe. At that moment, it became clear to me that I was now a father. I leaped for joy. I can remember hugging her and rubbing her stomach. We were both ecstatic!

We later revealed my wife's pregnancy to our immediate family & friends and later to our social media family. All of whom celebrated with us, the newly discovered fetus that was about to bring us tremendous joy.

Chapter Two

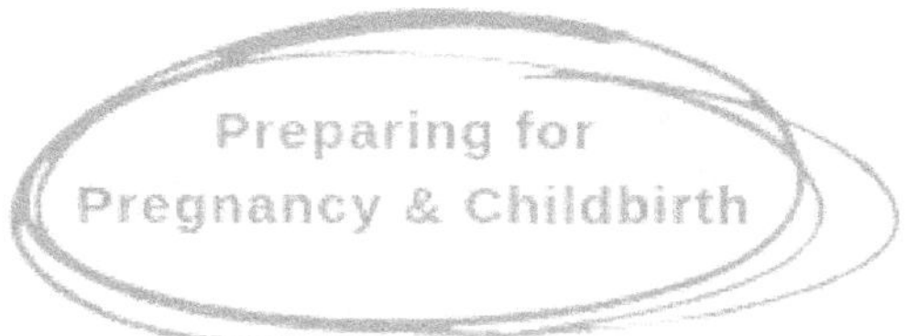

" The joy of conception is an important element to enjoy, but preparing for pregnancy & childbirth is another significant element that must be consistently applied.

Celebrating the conception & gender of our firstborn is a moment that will forever be engraved in our hearts. However, after all the celebration, it was time to begin preparing for the duration of our pregnancy and childbirth.

Open Doors

If you, then, though you are evil, know how to give good gifts to your children, how much more will your Father in heaven give good gifts to those who ask him.

- Matthew 7:11 (NIV)

For many, the process of preparing for the arrival of a newborn commonly begins with a focus on all the things that were never achieved before conception. Things such as a car, a better paying job, a house, or an apartment. After moving to the states, Tianka & I lived with her aunt for a year. Our deepest desire and constant prayer were that God would open a door for us to live within our own space. We prayed relentlessly for an apartment, but God kept saying, "No, not yet." When we tried moving against God's will and timing, He closed all doors. No matter how we tried, somehow, there would be a sudden spike in the prices for an apartment rental.

Suddenly, a couple of days after learning about Tianka's pregnancy, God led us to an apartment. The community was beautiful, peaceful, the price was affordable, and the location between our jobs was perfect. We had public transportation at our fingertips. Our church, major grocery stores, and shopping centers were within proximity to our home. To top it off, we had all the necessary help to move our stuff.

It was then I realized that our baby came with a shower of blessings and open doors. We didn't have a car; however, we had several offers from people who God had sent to purchase a car for us. Looking back, these were things that we both worked hard for and applied our faith in asking God to grant us, and He did.

My point is, don't start your preparation process with a heavy focus on all the things that you or you and your partner never achieved individually or collectively before conceiving. Whether it's a car, a new job, a promotion, a house, or an apartment, our Heavenly-Father knows exactly what you need even before you ask him! He will provide for you. Just trust Him. I believe that God has already sent your new bundle of joy with his/her blessings and open doors.

The Importance of Creating a Birth Plan

Like everything else in life, you need a plan. Creating a birth plan will force you to educate yourself about childbirth so that you're able to make informed decisions throughout pregnancy, labor, and delivery. Although the natural course of labor and delivery will take place, your birth plan will help protect you and your child's health and safety by making decisions on your behalf as you endure the mental, physical, and emotional roller coaster ride of labor and delivery.

Your birth plan will also be one of the most important documents that will outline and determine the outcome of almost 65 percent, if not more of your birthing experience. It will determine how you plan for worst-case scenarios and how you want them handled. Throughout my wife's childbirth experience, I learned that every birth is unique. Therefore, every mother's birth plan must be uniquely orchestrated to meet their heart's desires. This unique birth plan will help you to communicate your desires and wishes to those caring for you during labor, delivery, and after the birth of your baby. More importantly, your birth plan will help you to determine the type of birth you would like to have; and in some cases, your birth plan helps you to prepare a plan B in the case where a mother's plan A has failed.

Tianka's Birth Plan

Our firmest belief is that God created humans to be fruitful. As of such, He created the human body to bring forth children naturally. Therefore, Tianka wanted a natural childbirth. We did a thorough research about modern science's method of handling labor and delivery, and we wanted no part in it. We discovered how some medical professionals dishonored the natural flow of labor and delivery and had created their artificial flow that's jammed with trickery and intimidating factors. Such intimidating factors were applied to make what was meant to be a natural, unnatural, and expensive process. We also learned about the negative effects of the common drugs (Pitocin and Epidural) that are used in modern science's labor and delivery procedure. As such, Tianka wanted an un-medicated natural home birth. That became our plan A.

The Importance of a Birth kit

" Our birth kit is synonymous with a first aid kit. It's a collection of supplies and equipment that should be readily available to be used in unforeseen circumstances.

What if you were to go into labor when you're least expecting to, are you prepared? It's profoundly said that there's no reason to have a "plan B" because it only distracts you from your "plan A." *However, what if you planned for a home-birth and it turns out that you're transferred to the hospital; is your birth kit equipped with all the necessary supplies to sustain you?*

Tianka and I only planned for a supernatural home birth. *Have you ever heard of it?* If you haven't, here's a brief definition of what it's about "A supernatural childbirth is the childbirth that occurs with the supernatural intervention of God. Supernatural childbirth is usually pain-free and has little to no obstacles. The concept of supernatural childbirth derived from a belief that Jesus has redeemed us from the burden of the Old Testament law, which states, "Then he said to the woman, "I will sharpen the pain of your pregnancy, and in pain, you will give birth. And you will desire to control your husband, but he will rule over you." *Genesis 3:16*. However, through the life, death, and resurrection of Christ, we attained freedom from the burden of the law. See *Galatians 3:13*. This means that we have redemption in all areas of our life once we have a personal relationship with Christ. When people suggested that we ought to be open-minded to other birthing methods, we created a mental block.

We thought they were consciously as well as unconsciously trying to inject fear and negativity into our plan A. We believed that preparing for something else other than what we believed and were asking God for was an indication that we had a lack of faith. Hmm... Boy, was I wrong! Tianka experienced all three childbirth methods, and our birth kit was only prepared to sustain us for one method of delivery—a supernatural home birth. When we realized that Tianka had to be transferred to the hospital, it took us a long time to put together a birth kit that would sustain us both at the hospital. After arriving at the hospital, Tianka and I realized that after all the packing that we had done, we still didn't pack adequate supplies. Especially not for the seven days admission that was ahead of us.

Are you or you and your partner planning for the unpredictable? I hope so. After Geor'nyah was born and admitted to the neonatal intensive care unit (NICU), I had to rush back to our apartment and pack two suitcases.

Whether you're planning for a home or hospital birth, a birth kit should always be prepared for your method of childbirth. If you're planning for a home birth, I recommend that you arrange a birth kit for your home birth and an additional birth kit just in case you have to be transferred to the hospital. Doing this will ensure that you are prepared, not only for medical treatment but also allows you to bring a slice of your home's tranquility to the hospital's environment.

In the coming chapters, I will talk more about the importance of a birth kit and share important things to consider when creating a birth kit.

The Importance of Birth Class

Before Tianka and I got enrolled in an independent birth class, we watched a lot of videos and read a lot of blog articles, and I mean – A LOT! I acquired so much information through videos, blog articles, and hearing other couples' testimony that I thought that taking a birth class was over-rated. My entire perspective changed after Tianka and I got enrolled in a birth class. As my wife's main support system, I learned a lot of theoretical information as well as practical exercises that prepared me for the big day. I got an in-depth training on breathing techniques that would help her to breathe properly through her contractions. I learned the importance of taking charge of our birthing environment by eradicating unwanted energy from people. I learned the different stages of labor and how to identify when my wife transitioned through the various stages of labor. We learned about pain management & how to manage early labor pain, comfortable labor positions, how your partner can help you during labor, and when to call your doctor or midwife. Overall, everything I learned throughout our birth class prepared me to be mentally and emotionally sound for what was to come.

Tianka and I learned of a few mothers that went into childbirth uninformed and unprepared, and the experience is never as smooth sailing as it would have been if they were educated on childbirth. Therefore, please don't procrastinate about getting enrolled in a birth class. A birth class will build your confidence, and provide your partner with evidence-based information that will help prepare you both for a positive birth experience regardless of how labor unfolds.

In the coming chapters, you will learn more about childbirth classes, and how to select the birth class that's right for you.

Chapter Three

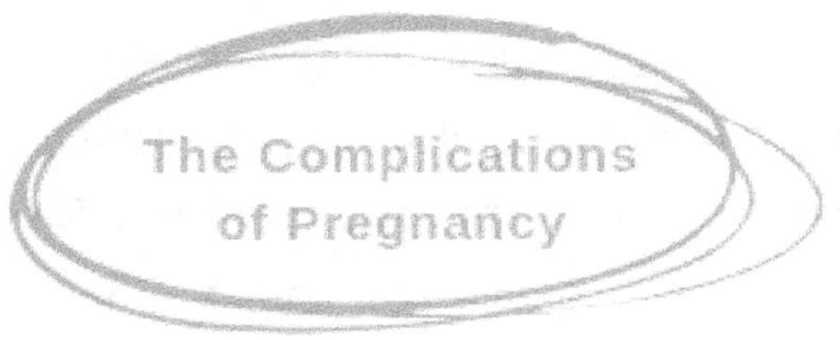

" *When your body starts developing complications, know that you aren't failing, it's not your fault, and you are strong enough to endure the many severe pregnancy complications.*

Tianka's Battle with Gestational Diabetes

Gestational diabetes occurs when a pregnant woman's body is unable to make and use all the insulin it needs for pregnancy. Without adequate insulin, glucose (sugar) cannot leave the blood and be changed into energy.

In Tianka's case, at 30 something weeks, her body was producing very little insulin.   She had a lot of sugar stored in her blood and nothing to help diminish it. Our midwife explained that if Tianka's gestational diabetes weren't treated properly, then all the stored-up sugar in her body would be passed onto her baby, giving her baby more glucose than what she needs to grow and develop. The extra sugar (glucose) also meant that our baby would have more energy, being that this energy cannot be physically expressed, all of that energy would be stored as fat and possibly lead to macrosomia or a fat baby. Our midwife further explained that babies with macrosomia face potential health problems such as damage to their shoulders during, and are also at a higher risk for developing breathing problems. Babies with excess insulin also become at risk for obesity and childhood diabetes earlier on in their life.

Treating Gestational Diabetes

To effectively treat gestational diabetes, Tianka had to make an immediate decision to change her diet to protect our baby and herself from all the potential dangers of gestational diabetes. A sudden restriction was placed on high-carbohydrates and a high-sugar diet. We bought a glucose monitor to help manage and determine how much concentration of glucose was in her blood after each meal.

She had to sacrifice her favorite foods, but it was worth it. The diet change kept her sugar level at a healthy level. It worked so well that she developed a routine and no longer needed the glucose monitor to determine the amount of glucose in her blood. She just knew what to eat and the portion size. If you aren't troubled with insulin resistance, it's still important to be cognizant of your sugar intake. Too much sugar creates a spur in a baby's heart rate, which has negative consequences for the baby. In the coming chapters, I will go in-depth about a diet plan that will help you with getting your blood glucose levels in the best shape if you are faced with the challenge of gestational diabetes. I will also share more on its effects on mothers and their babies.

Finding Out Our Baby was in a Posterior Position

Daily movement and exercise is what's needed to help place a baby in its proper position for delivery

During Tianka's 35 weeks checkup, our midwife discovered that our baby wasn't inducted in her proper position. She was positioned head down with her back on the right side of Tianka's stomach. Medical science defines this as an occipital-posterior position. After learning of this, our midwife started ranting about all the negative outcomes that could result from this situation. Like a broken record, she kept reiterating all the potential adverse outcomes. Soon enough, our midwife's negative impact overwhelmed Tianka. Thoughts of having a breech baby immediately flashed through her mind, as well as the possibility of having to do an emergency cesarean section. While our midwife was babbling away, I had to grab hold of my mind. I began reciting encouraging scriptures in my head to maintain my sanity. As soon as I got myself together, I started whispering encouraging scriptures over my wife. For a moment, it was effective.

But Tianka soon melted into tears. She was extremely fatigued from dealing with her boss at work. An employee had resigned, and they were short-staffed. After working back to back over-time at her job, Tianka was exhausted. On the day of her midwife check-up, Tianka was working to fulfill her regular role as well as to fulfill the role of the employee who had resigned. She was overworked, nauseous, and needed to use the bathroom. When Tianka asked her boss to cover for her so she could get a bathroom break and to have lunch, her boss replied, "I have to go home and feed my dog." Her boss made it clear that the well-being of her dog was more important than the well-being of a child and my wife.

That day our midwife knew the drama that my wife had dealt with at work before coming into our appointment. Nonetheless, she thought it is wise to add more fuel to a burning flame. We understood that it's our midwife's job to inspect and report to us any potential risks associated with Tianka's pregnancy. However, it's not what was said that was discomforting; it was how she delivered the message. What was also discomforting is that our midwife appeared to be more emotionally unsound than us.

As a professional, I wish she would have maintained composure. Especially since she knew Tianka was battling with a few pregnancy complications, and stress at work. In the words of *Matthew 6:34* - today's troubles are enough for today. As a professional, I wish she didn't exaggerate the situation. I wish she kept her emotions concealed, simply because we weren't paying her to express how she felt, we were paying her to assist us based on her knowledge and experience.

In the coming chapters, I will state some important tips and advice that will be useful in helping you screen & choose the best health–care provider to embark with you and your baby on your nine months journey.

How Tianka Rotated A Posterior Baby

At 35 weeks, a baby should begin rotating to assume a head down, feet up position with his or her back towards the front of their mother's stomach - this is called the occipital-anterior position. It allows a baby to glide in and out of a woman's pelvis easily during pregnancy and labor. Medical research has shown that the main benefit of the anterior position is that pregnant mothers are less likely to have an emergency cesarean section. Medical research also states that mothers are more likely to have quicker labor and delivery that require less pain-relief drugs.

If a baby isn't fully situated in an occipital-anterior position, the power of contractions and the movement of the baby's feet will sometimes help with rotating the baby from an occipital-posterior position into an occipital-anterior position. However, the ratio of that happening is a 50/50 chance. We weren't going to take that risk, especially when there are exercises that can be done to help correct the occipital-posterior position of a child.

Tianka and I thought about firing our midwife and transfer to another health-care provider. However, being that Tianka was already 35 weeks pregnant, it was a hard and risky decision to make. It meant that we had to do the necessary research to find a new health-care provider, have Tianka's files transferred to that new health-care provider, undergo a series of new ultrasounds, etc. to educate our new midwife on where we were at in our journey. As you can see, it would require a lot of time, energy, and resources that we didn't have. Therefore, we opted to overlook our midwife's unprofessional behavior and trust her expertise in moving forward. We embarked on a clean slate which involved moving forward with solutions. Tianka did thorough research and began applying a few old midwives' theories along with applying our midwife's recommendation. After selecting the right exercises for Tianka, she went ahead and applied them. We discovered that left-side sleeping is the best sleeping position for pregnant women, especially if your baby had become comfortable with living inside the womb in a posterior position. So, I had to ensure that Tianka was always sleeping on her left side along with other exercises that would help encourage the baby to change her position.

We also did a lot of walking daily; I ensured that whenever Tianka is sitting down, she had good posture by sitting up straight or by sitting a little bit forward and that her knees were lower than her hips.

When Tianka's sister came to visit, we used water and gravity to our benefit by taking Tianka to the pool. We helped her to float on her stomach. Doing this helped to pull the baby out of her current position and forced her to fall at the front of Tianka's tummy and further down her pelvis. These were a few of the methods that we applied based on our midwife's recommendation.

Did they work? Absolutely! In the coming chapters, I share effective and efficient baby repositioning exercises that will help you reposition your posterior baby into an anterior position.

Tianka's Challenge of Being Pregnant with Polycystic Ovarian Syndrome (PCOS)

Polycystic ovarian syndrome (PCOS) is a common health problem among women that struggle with an imbalance of reproductive hormones. Women with PCOS usually have high levels of insulin, or male hormones known as 'androgens,' or sometimes both. The cause of PCOS is unknown; however, insulin resistance is thought to be the main problem for women diagnosed with PCOS. PCOS often causes missed or irregular menstrual periods. Irregular menstrual periods often lead to infertility (inability to get pregnant). PCOS is one of the most common causes of infertility in women. Women with PCOS are also known to develop cysts on their ovaries. Based on Tianka's experience with being pregnant with PCOS, there are a couple of things that I learned from research such as women with this health problem are at a higher risk for pregnancy and delivery complications.

Delivery complications commonly involve extremely slow dilation and weak or inconsistent contractions during labor. Women pregnant with PCOS usually require medical interventions such as Pitocin (a synthetic version of the natural oxytocin that a woman's body produces.) It's used as a medication to kick start heavy and consistent contractions. Women pregnant with PCOS may also need a cesarean section (c-section). These outcomes are usually as a result of the hormone imbalance and a pregnant woman's body not being able to generate a build-up of adequate hormones to deliver a child successfully.

One of the biggest potholes that women with PCOS try to avoid along their pregnancy journey is hitting the pothole of having a miscarriage during their first trimester. While every pregnant woman is extremely cautious about making it through their first trimester of pregnancy, there is a three-fold increase in having a miscarriage in early pregnancy compared to women without PCOS. Therefore, getting past the first trimester for a pregnant woman with PCOS is a great sigh of relief. As for Tianka, when she found out that she was pregnant, she always had a lingering fear at the back of her mind about having a miscarriage. The first trimester of her pregnancy was a period in which she was waiting to exhale. So much fear surrounded her pregnancy that she was hesitant to announce her pregnancy publicly until her second trimester. That's when she felt most confident. After she overcame the battering fear of having a miscarriage in the first trimester, she had to contend with the fear of having a premature birth in her second trimester.

One theory regarding miscarriage in women diagnosed with polycystic ovarian syndrome is that the occurrence is related to elevated insulin levels. Insulin resistance (IR) occurs when a woman's blood cells begin to reject insulin. This results in the inability of a woman's cells to convert blood sugar into energy. Having high insulin levels can result in increased blood clotting at the interface between the uterine lining and the placenta, which could lead to placental insufficiency. It can also lead to a failure of the placenta to supply nutrients to the fetus and remove toxic wastes. The result can be a miscarriage because it has the potential of affecting the quality of the egg and the function of the reproductive organs.

Another major pothole is that pregnant women with PCOS are at risk of developing gestational diabetes. Studies show that gestational diabetes is seen in about four (4) percent of all pregnancies but is seen more commonly in women with PCOS. Unfortunately, Tianka was a part of that four (4) percent. Tianka's battle with gestational diabetes, PCOS, a baby in a posterior position, and carpal tunnel syndrome has beaten her down to her knees one too many times. Nonetheless, she decided not to complain; rather, she rose to the occasion. If you are struggling with PCOS, gestational diabetes, a baby in a posterior position, or with any other pregnancy ailment that's unmentioned in this book, then she wants to encourage you to be strong and remain firm in your faith. Instead of focusing on all the possible negative outcomes, focus more on the positive solutions to every challenge that may take a swing at your pregnancy. Despite the increased risks, a lot of women go on to have normal and healthy babies.

Tianka's Battle with Carpal Tunnel Syndrome

Carpal tunnel syndrome (CTS) is a common issue that most pregnant women experience. It occurs when a fluid by the name of Oedmema has been built up in the tissues of the wrist. Once the fluid builds up, it compresses against the median nerve in your hand (s) and fingers, which causes tingles and numbness. Tianka's battle with carpal tunnel syndrome began in her third trimester. Her symptoms included numbness, tingling, swelling, and pain in both hands. She also lost her fingers' ability to grip things tightly. Partaking in any activity that required her to use her hands or fingers was painful and extremely difficult.

Treating Carpal Tunnel Syndrome

Tianka's remedy for minimizing and coping with the effects of carpal tunnel syndrome includes a wrist splinting/brace. Since frequent bending of your wrist adds loads of pressure on the median nerve found in your wrist, using a wrist splint prevented her wrist from bending by keeping her hand in a neutral position. Lucky for Tianka, using a wrist splint was the only remedy that she needed to treat her CTS. It alleviated the swelling, pain, tingling, and numbness in both of her hands. Once she gave birth, all of the systems slowly died away.

Finding a remedy that treats carpal tunnel syndrome is not a one size fits all. Therefore, I've added additional remedies that may help you to alleviate the effects of carpal tunnel syndrome. In the coming chapters, you'll learn more about these.

Chapter Four

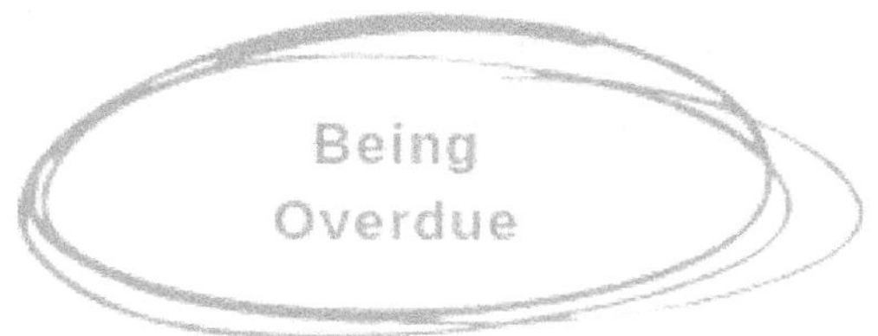

> **"** *Due dates are rarely accurate; they're only a medical prediction. Only the creator truly knows when your fetus was created. Although it's scary & nerve-racking, relax. Your baby will come on its own time.*

The word "Overdue" can be defined as not having arrived, happened, or been done by the expected time. However, when it comes to being pregnant and overdue, there is no scientific evidence that can truly articulate the reason for the unpunctual arrival of a child. In Tianka's case, her due date had passed, and this breathed a lot of anxiety and frustration. When asked about the matter of being overdue, Tianka was assured by her midwife not to worry because this was her first pregnancy

& most babies tend to arrive late in the mother's first pregnancy. Tianka was also told that her due date might have been miscalculated, possibly due to confusion over the exact date of the start of her last menstrual cycle. Amid our baby being overdue, many medical observations were considered, all of which had the potential of being a suitable candidate for our case. Although we both were grateful to have a baby on the way, we learned that pregnancy is a bed of roses; it's beautiful; however, once you lay in it, you'll realize that it also has thorns. Those thorns are the complications of pregnancy that Tianka and other moms experience along the way. The backache, mood swings, skin pigmentation, nausea, vomiting, diet changes, being pregnant with PCOS and dealing with the crippling fear of having a miscarriage, premature birth, gestational diabetes, the worry of being overdue, trying to correct the occipital-posterior position that her baby was in, and also dealing with challenges that came with her job were officially unbearable.

On the matter of being overdue, Tianka was also becoming perturbed about the health of our child & her body's capability to withstand the possible dangers of growing a child inside of her that long without being susceptible to the consequences of our daughter passing meconium (feces) inside her.

Tianka was now over 41 weeks pregnant, and all that she had been experiencing were Braxton hicks contractions—otherwise known as practice contractions. Being over 41 weeks in, and still, no baby was a scary process for Tianka. If a woman's pregnancy lasts longer than 42 weeks (294 days), it's called a prolonged pregnancy. Although most babies and moms remain healthy throughout a prolonged pregnancy, studies show that a small number of babies often die unexpectedly while they are still inside the womb or shortly after their birth. Studies also show that the number of babies who are stillborn or who die shortly after birth gradually increases between 39 and 42 weeks. That, coupled together with the risk of fetal distress and knowing that stillbirth rises steeply after 42 weeks, particularly for women expecting their first baby, made Tianka felt like the odds were against her. And I must admit, I thought so too.

I felt bad for my wife; I watched her as she read blog articles, and watched YouTube videos all day and night, seeking information, comfort, and community. I gave her all the mental, emotional, and spiritual support that I had to offer. However, she needed to hear from other women, especially women, who were overdue. There were mornings and nights when sniffles & tears awakened me. She would turn and ask me the question, "*Is Geor'nyah and I going to be okay?*" I would respond, "Absolutely, you both are going to be fine, it's all going to happen according to God's perfect timing, and when it does, He's gonna take care of you both." If she asked me that question a hundred times, 50 percent of the time, I was struggling to believe it myself, and I was crying on the inside as well.

Nonetheless, I showed no negative emotions. I would wait until Tianka was fully asleep at night, and I would cry my doubts and frustrations out of my heart. It's not that I was a liar, but I couldn't allow her to see me shattered when she's already torn apart. I had to keep it together or appear to be. If I were to be humorous, I'd faked it until we made it through the storm.

Tianka Inducing Labor

Inducing labor can be defined as the stimulation of uterine contractions during pregnancy before labor begins on its own to achieve a vaginal birth. Leading up to 42 weeks, Tianka frantically searched the internet for ways to induce labor naturally. We applied a series of natural inducing methods that were suggested by her midwife. After trying all of the natural inducing methods that our midwife deemed safe, Tianka still hadn't gone into labor. We couldn't believe it. She worked assiduously in applying each method, but still, all that she experienced were Braxton Hicks contractions. It was disappointing. Once again, Tianka was in between meltdowns. What was also frustrating for her was that she heard the success stories of many women who tried these natural inducing methods. Please don't misunderstand us, she's happy for the mothers that tried natural inducing methods and received positive results, but as a result of all the pregnancy complications she was dealing with, Tianka began to question if her body was inferior. I had to reassure her that her body was perfect; however, whether it's a medical or natural induction method, every woman's body and pregnancy will respond differently to inducing methods. Therefore, no method is guaranteed to induce you to labor.

During another midwife check-up, Tianka was given a natural medication known as black cohosh to help ripen her cervix. She was scheduled for another ultrasound in two (2) days. The results of that ultrasound would determine the baby's movement, weight, size, and position. The results would also help to determine whether

Tianka was suitable to induce labor medically or if she could wait a couple more days beyond her due date without medical or surgical intervention.

Myself, my wife, and mid-wife re-visited all the risks that were associated with Tianka being overdue. We agreed that if Tianka didn't go into labor over the weekend (between Saturday, June 16 and Sunday, June 17, 2018), then Tianka would have to visit her back-up doctor on Tuesday, June 19, 2018, for a consultation, another ultrasound, and possibly to induce labor.

Chapter Five

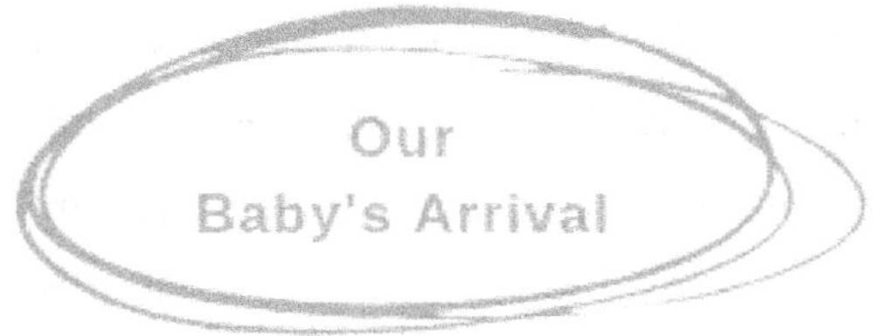

On Saturday, June 16, 2018, at 4:30 am, Tianka was awakened by the feeling of wet fluid flowing between her legs. Feeling both startled and excited, she woke me up! "Babe, Babe!" she shouted twice. By the tone of her voice, I already figured that her water might have broke. I rolled over, pulled back the sheets, and looked at her. "*What's going on?*" I asked. "I think my water just broke." She replied. She wanted to use the bathroom, so I jumped out of bed and escorted her to the bathroom.

Suddenly, a burst of clear brownish fluid dispensed from her body and crashed against our bathroom floor. We both looked at each other in such amazement! The look on our face was almost as if we had gotten a million bucks. We both thought, "It's finally happening!" Everything felt surreal! I burst out in uncontainable laughter! I sprinted to our living room to wake up her sister, who came from New York to baby watch with us. I thought to myself, "All the birthing exercises, long daily walks, and natural inducing methods that we applied had finally paid off."

Tianka's sister came two weeks in advance to be a part of Tianka's natural home birth. When labor kept delaying, her sister constantly extended her stay at the risk of losing her job.

Making Final Preparations

I learned that the best way to keep a pregnant woman calm during labor is to create an environment that stimulates the five human senses—hearing, sight, smell, taste, and touch. To stimulate her hearing, I had several playlists filled with instrumentals, sounds of nature, scripture declarations, and gospel music. I also had positive affirmations to encourage her through labor. To stimulate her smell, I ensured that the environment and everything in it had a fresh and clean aroma, preferably the scent of fresh linen. I also had her favorite scented candles — eucalyptus mint, and peppermint oil to pour into our diffuser. To stimulate her taste buds, our birth team and I ensured she had all her favorite snacks and food. Not just any food, but food that would replenish her. For beverages, I had several bottles of coconut water from freshly chopped coconuts (You can get this at local or international farmer's market) to keep her hydrated and to give her the electrolytes that she needs for energy and recovery. For physical touch, I knew her pressure points, and just how to utilize the techniques that I learned from our birthing class and masseuse. Heat provides relaxation to sore and aching muscles and aggravated nerves. So I placed several washcloths in our electric slow cooker to keep them warm. If she felt hot and needed to cool down, I soaked a few other washcloths in water and placed inside our refrigerator to be frozen. All of these were prepared in advance to stimulate all her five (5) senses, give her a sense of external order, strengthen her confidence, and to silence any whisper of fear or feelings of anxiety.

Contractions

> *Labor is like a marathon that if run like a race,*
> *you risk being burned out.*

In the early stages of labor, Tianka's contractions weren't as painful. They were between 30 and 55 seconds long and were 15-20 minutes apart. As the day progressed, her contractions intensified. I applied all the coping techniques we were taught in childbirth class to help pace Tianka's energy usage and breathing so she could endure this marathon to the end. After a few hours had passed, Tianka called her midwife and gave a brief update. Our midwife lived 10 minutes away from us. We also called her aunt, who later came over with her daughter, Tianka's cousin. They were all a part of Tianka's birth support team and were there to provide mental, emotional, and spiritual upliftment. They were also there to help Tianka through this marathon in whatever capacity.

During our midwife's first visit, Tianka was nowhere close to being a centimeter dilated. She asked if Tianka had her bloody show or if her mucus plug was release yet; with Tianka's response being "No, not yet," our midwife advised us to brace ourselves because this could be a long labor. She did other check-ups and discovered that the baby's heart rate was perfectly normal. She also informed us that the baby's position was a bit off again and that the baby's head had slightly slipped out of her pelvis. She mentioned that during the process of checking Tianka's cervix and reaching for the baby's head, the crown of the baby's head slowly floated away. Without trying to conceal her emotions, we noticed an instant look of fear on our midwife's face.

She suggested that Tianka do a couple of exercises to position the baby further into her pelvis to promote a faster and natural dilation. The goal was to get and keep the position of the baby's head deeper within Tianka's pelvis. That way, the constant force of each contraction would apply the pressure of the baby's head against her cervix and help with effacement and dilation. The first exercise that our midwife performed on Tianka was called the rebozo. The rebozo method involved Tianka being on her hands and knees while our midwife stood over her and placed a rebozo shawl around her stomach and moved it in a sifting motion. This technique is known to provide relaxation without the intervention of synthetic drugs. However, our midwife applied this method for the sole purpose of the rebozo technique, which is to create space for the baby inside the tummy by relaxing tight uterine ligaments and abdominal muscles and helped the baby rotate and get into the best position for labor. Tianka's reaction to this old Mexican technique was the opposite of relaxation and comfort. Instead, she was in deep pain. Tears marched from her eyes as she screamed her way through this session. She lost composure, and her breathing became out of rhythm. It was hard watching her endure such pain. However, I remained level-headed. I got down on my knees and helped her regain her correct breathing pattern. At that moment, my words of affirmation that I prepared beforehand to stimulate her sense of hearing came in handy. I spoke those words softly in her ears while tears climbed down her cheeks. At the end of the rebozo session, the technique accomplished its core purpose. The rebozo was followed by another exercise which involved Tianka leaning against a wall in an upright position to do a few reps of pelvic rock. Pelvic rock is used by women in labor to help them focus during contractions and assist with moving the baby down into the birth canal. This too was agonizing for Tianka simply because it was forcing the pressure of the baby on her cervix. She described the sensation as a foot banging consistently against a door. She stated that at times, she felt as if the baby's head was piercing through her anus. The upright pelvic position was followed by Tianka squatting/sitting on her birth ball with her legs spread apart. This exercise was suggested as another method to relax her pelvic muscles and widen her pelvis.

She gently rocked side to side, along with bouncing at different intervals. The aim was to use gravity to bring the pressure of the baby's head down onto her cervix to encourage dilation. Bear in mind, Tianka was doing all of these exercises amid her contractions. It was rigorous! The look on her face said it all, and by the strength of her groan, I could tell that it was beyond difficult for her. Our midwife's theory was that by performing all of these exercises amid her contractions, the contractions would complement her exercises by adding force to propel the baby downwards. After doing all of this, more fluids came gushing down.

During labor, you always want to know if your baby is showing signs of fetal distress. Therefore, we asked for periodic heart rate checkups. Our midwife's second heart rate check showed that the baby's heart rate was once again normal. Knowing that your baby's heartbeat is normal brings true comfort and peace. It was God's way of letting us know that our baby had the peace of Christ that passes human comprehension. And that gave Tianka the courage and tenacity to press on in labor. Before leaving, our midwife encouraged Tianka to be less active and instructed her to lie down on her left side with a pillow between her legs. She left and said that she would be back between one (1) and three (3) hours and advised us to keep her updated.

After 12 hours of labor, Tianka was only 1 cm dilated.

2 Centimeters Dilated

After our midwife left the house, Tianka slept lightly for a few minutes. After waking up, we went for a short walk. We knew that walking would use gravity to pull the baby further down and put pressure on the cervix to encourage dilation. During our walk, she had quite a few contractions; we continued with our midwife's suggested method, which was to have her squat during each contraction. This too was rigorous; however, Tianka was willing to endure any exercise method to help her dilate faster. After a short five minutes walk and a couple of squats, she stepped up a staircase that was at our apartment complex, skipping a stair each time, and then we went back home. We waited a couple more hours before calling our midwife again. After calling her, she said that she would be there soon. Some time had passed, and we didn't see her. After calling her again, she told us that she had just finished delivering another baby and was doing the baby's measurement. Tianka and I were shocked! We understood that if we were at the hospital, the doctors would have done the same thing and would have attended to another mother in labor. However, we were more stunned at the fact that she didn't communicate during her last house visit that she was leaving to assist another birth. That made us thought of all the possible things that could have gone wrong while she was at another person's birth. In my opinion, this was extremely reckless.

At a hospital, there's a heart-rate monitor to monitor the baby's heart rate. This lets the doctors, as well as the parents, know that the baby is healthy. During our home birth, our midwife only had a basic portable fetal heart rate monitor. It worked. I'm not discrediting its ability. However, she took her heart rate monitor with her to deliver somebody else's child that could have taken a long time to be delivered. We weren't even left with an assistant midwife to do periodic check-ups. I mean, the least she could have done was to tell us, so in case of an emergency, we would be prepared to exercise other options. To this day, I thank God that our normalcy didn't break out in an emergent situation while she was away.

Another 40 minutes to an hour had gone before she finally arrived at our apartment. It took only a glance for us to realize that whatever bad experience she had at the birth, she had taken it to our house and was about to inject all that bad energy into our environment. She looked more exhausted and irritable than Tianka, who was laboring for more than 16 hours. Each checkup that she did was followed-up by a brief explanation that became repetitive and was sprinkled with smart disrespectful comments. She never displayed a caring and understanding attitude. She is an experienced midwife, but she lacked emotional composure and professional tact. Everyone, including Tianka, wanted to snap at her. However, we figured that would be adding fuel to a burning flame.

At 8:38 PM, she checked Tianka's cervix. After hours of intense contractions and exercises, Tianka was only 2 cm dilated. Tianka was in great disbelief! She thought that she would have at least been 3 cm dilated.

Our midwife explained that Tianka's cervix was thinner than before; therefore, we can expect things to speed up. She also checked the baby's heart rate, and it was perfect. She stayed with us for a while and later left to grab a cup of coffee and to regroup.

The Power of Our Support Team

Words are inadequate to explain how supportive our family was throughout the entire experience. They were helping us from the moment they arrived at our apartment. Tianka's aunt was always in the kitchen, fixing us something to eat while her sister and her cousin ensured that the environment was peaceful. When Tianka needed something from the store, they were both available. As the night grew older, they continued to extend their hand of support. They realized that I was exhausted. I was with Tianka the entire time, ensuring that she was relaxed, breathing correctly, timing her contractions, massaging her, applying pressure to her lower back, helping her with her exercises, rubbing her tummy, providing bathroom assistance, and encouraging her. Please don't get me wrong; I'm not complaining. I fully embrace and submit to my responsibilities as her husband and the father to our child. However, at this point, I needed to at least close my eyes for five minutes.

After several yawns, I looked at the clock, and it was 10 pm. Everyone knew how tired they were and that things were only warming up. So, we created a schedule for the remaining duration of the night and the early stages of the morning. We each took shifts for sleeping and eating.

At around 11 pm, Tianka's contractions were coming back to back. As soon as a contraction ended, another one started. They were so intense that we could see her stomach moving in a wave-like motion. We could also see the baby's movement during each contraction. At this point, Tianka began using the toilet sitting technique. Toilet sitting may not sound too welcoming; however, like walking and squatting, this technique will help to relax your pelvic muscles and get gravity on your side as it forces the baby's head onto your cervix to speed up dilation. Of all the dilation techniques that Tianka had done, she described the toilet sitting as being the most difficult and painful method. While using this method, she stated that a heavy load of pressure from the baby's head came crashing down on her rectum. She said that it was so much pressure for her that it blurred the line between "pressure" and "pain." After sitting down, it was hard for her to get up off the toilet seat. On top of that, she had to get up fast enough before another contraction would start.

At midnight, she called her midwife and explained how intense her contractions became. They were lasting between 60 and 95 seconds and were 3-8 minutes apart. Her contractions were closer together, and she had less time to walk around. We thought that surely Tianka had further dilated and that she was getting closer to active labor. So, we asked her midwife to come in and perform a cervix check. She began explaining the possible dangers of frequent cervix checks and that it could cause unwanted infections. She said that she was going to be at our house in 30 minutes, and if Tianka hadn't dilated any further, she would have to be hospitalized. Hearing the word "hospital" brought chills to our bodies. I looked at Tianka, and I could see the fear in her eyes. It made us knew that this situation was on the verge of transitioning into an extreme experience.

Nonetheless, we prayed and believed that God would turn things around in our favor. Both Tianka and I had family and friends back home, praying on our behalf. We wholeheartedly believed that if we agreed together in forbidding a hospital birth, or a c-section, then it would have been forbidden by our Father in Heaven. We also believed that if we agreed and permitted a natural home birth-the way, God intended a woman to bring forth a child, then it would have been granted.

You may be reading this and thinking that's foolish faith, and we should've started preparing for a transition to the hospital. Well, the cold truth is that you're right! We should have foreseen that based on all the signs, but in all transparency, it's hard to discover which path to take when your vision is clouded by fear. Tianka feared to have a c-section so much that she despised it. I too feared and despised the thought of seeing my wife sliced open to get a baby out of her. In addition to our fears, both Tianka and her mom had a terrible c-section story. One which resulted in the death of a child. As a result of the many fear that we had, we failed to remember that God's providence would see Tianka through, even if it meant that she had to undergo a c-section.

Blinded by Fear

It was becoming more evident that Tianka needed to be hospitalized. However, the fear that we both shared fueled our faith to remain hopeful that God was about to turn things around, even though God was making it obvious that we needed to be transferred to the hospital. Looking back on that day, we both realized that we missed so many of God's cues. It's safe to say that our faith was fueled by fear, and our eyes were blinded by fear.

The last time that Tianka spoke to her midwife, she told Tianka that she would return to the house in 30 minutes. However, our midwife showed up three (3) hours later. Her explanation for arriving that late was because she wanted to give my wife more time to dilate.

She checked Tianka's cervix and stated that she was three centimeters dilated. She reiterated that we should start considering the hospital. We called our support team into the bedroom and explained our midwife's prognosis. Suddenly, Tianka's sister froze up. She stood with her arms folded along with a strong look of disappointment, worry, and trauma. No matter how much we asked, "Are you okay?" she remained unresponsive. She too had believed God for a natural home-birth, so when Tianka's labor took another direction, her sister was stunned! We were all stunned! I did another time check, and it was 4:30 a.m. on Sunday, June 17. This marked 24 hours of intense labor. Once again, our midwife checked the baby's heart rate, and it was perfect. She made herself a bed on our couch and decided to stay at our house. She explained that she had assisted women who labored beyond 24-hours, and they had a successful natural home birth. She explained further that once the baby's heart rate is normal, then Tianka is fit to continue in labor. That sparked some optimism, and so we held onto that. Tianka's mom was tuned in via Skype. She, along with my sister, kept suggesting that we prepare for a hospital transfer; however, Tianka decided to continue laboring at home.

Hospital Transfer

Tianka had her final cervix check at 2:00 p.m., and she was still 3 centimeters dilated. On average, it took Tianka 6-8 hours to be a centimeter dilated. According to her midwife, Tianka's dilation had slowed down and became non-progressive. It was also evident that meconium (stool) was in Tianka's amniotic fluid. This meant that the baby had a bowel movement before or during labor. This also meant that the baby might have been stressed. It may also indicate that the baby has a mature gut which already started working (this is more common in overdue babies that are more neurologically mature). Whatever the reason, if the baby inhales the sticky meconium during her first breath, it would be difficult for her lungs to inflate. Tianka was also at risk because the longer meconium remains untreated inside of her, the more susceptible she becomes for an infection.

After 33 and a half hours of labor, Tianka felt weary, she felt like she couldn't go on. At this point, we could no longer be in enmity with the hospital and a prisoner to our fears. Our midwife immediately hopped on the phone and began making arrangements and completing the necessary forms for Tianka to be transferred to the care of her back-up doctor. She showered and got dressed while her aunt and I packed baby stuff, as well as clothing and toiletries for Tianka.

On our way to the hospital, I can remember the feeling of fear and defeat creeping into our hearts as we wondered and worried about what was ahead of us. As my wife's main support system, I remember saying to myself, this is no time to lose my focus. I encouraged myself according to *Deuteronomy 31:6 (NIV)*, which states, "Be strong and courageous. Do not be afraid or terrified because of them, for the Lord your God goes with you; he will never leave you nor forsake you." I gripped Tianka's hand and assured her that God's divine providence was with us and that he wasn't about to forsake us!

Upon arrival at the hospital, I remembered the sound and movement of the hospital doors and how wide they opened. I remembered the urgency of the seven nurses that approached us as we walked through those doors. It was like an episode of Grey's Anatomy in which surgery-hungry doctors yearned for the next patient so much that they waited eagerly for the next patient to walk through the hospital doors. While they had good intentions and were responding quickly to emergent situations, their responsiveness gave me the chills. I felt like I was taking my wife to the hospital to feed the surgical hunger of a bunch of doctors. A nurse took our information and then led us to our room, where she attached a heart rate monitor. She also checked Tianka and the baby's vital signs along with other procedures.

Surprisingly, the treatment that we received from our assigned nurse was a direct contrast to the poor care that Tianka received from her midwife. Our nurse was professional, but human enough to be compassionate towards my wife. She thoroughly explained each procedure that was going to take place. She was knowledgeable, experienced, and patient enough to answer all our questions. She was also honest about what Tianka's birthing experience was going to be like. Overall, our nurse went beyond the call of duty to ensure that Tianka was comfortable. Her hospitality gave us peace of mind and the confidence that was needed to trust the hospital staff. After Tianka's blood was withdrawn, she gave a urine sample for routine lab tests and later attached her IV (intravenous fluid line).

After Tianka's back-up doctor showed up, she explained to him what labor had been like thus far. Afterward, he did a cervix check, and Tianka was still 3 cm dilated. He then gave us two options and the possible outcome of each option. Option one involved Tianka taking Pitocin to speed up dilation by promoting stronger and consistent contractions. The potential positive outcome of "option one" is that Tianka may dilate further and give birth to a beautiful bouncing baby. The potential negative outcome of "option one" is that her cervix may remain unchanged, and she would have to undergo an emergency c-section. He explained that he had a past patient that labored beyond four days because her cervix was dilating extremely slow. However, she still gave birth to a healthy baby. He said that Tianka wasn't in a critical state and that the baby's heart rate was normal. This leads me to "option 2". "Option two" involved Tianka going back home to continue labor and see if there would be any cervical changes. This meant that we would have to visit him each day for however long it would take for her to be 5 cm dilated. The potential possible outcome was that Tianka would give birth to a healthy baby, or she would be re-admitted at the hospital for Pitocin and Epidural or for an emergency c-section.

He excused himself while we considered the best option. The idea of going back home sounded good at first because it meant that we still had the opportunity for a natural home birth. However, Tianka's mental, emotional, and physical condition wasn't fit to persevere without medical intervention. She stated although she hated the idea of synthetic drugs and their side-effects, she was just too tired and just could not go on. We also considered the possible dangers of the Meconium that was already released inside of her and felt that both Tianka and the baby would develop an infection as a result of the Meconium. Other secondary factors that we considered were that our support team had to return to work, her aunt and cousin lived one hour away, and her sister had to return to New York. We didn't have a vehicle to transport ourselves back and forth. Even if we did have a vehicle, we couldn't afford the daily charges to visit our back-up doctor at his office for him to test and monitor her progression. So, Tianka chose to stay at the hospital.

Suddenly, our reality started to speed up. Our nurse proceeded by explaining the steps that would follow. She ordered a bag of Pitocin and Epidural. By this time, I had managed to maintain external composure and tact regardless of the inner turmoil that was taking place. I had to, there were important decisions to make and important information that I had to be vigilant about to ensure that I understood and that I asked all the right questions. As soon as that phase had passed and all the documents were signed, I left the room. I walked the hallways hoping to clear my head and figure out how and when we ended up at the hospital.

Everything seemed to have fast-forwarded. I got tired of walking the hallways. I urgently needed to converse with God, so I found a bathroom, locked the door, and I unleashed all that fury that was inside my heart. In all honesty, I was angry! I felt like this was not what I asked from God. I was experiencing so many mixed emotions, many of which I couldn't understand. I was still in disbelief and utter shock that we had ended up in the hospital. In my conversation with God, I yelled: "This is not what we asked from you!" "We didn't prepare for this to happen!" "You didn't tell us that this was going to happen." " We asked you so many times, " *What was going to transpire?* "

"*What you wanted us to do?* " and you said

"Nothing! " *Why didn't you tell us we were going to end up at the hospital to experience what we were praying not to experience?* " "God, this doesn't make any sense!" I calmed down a little, and I said, "God, when Tianka and I found out we were pregnant, we prayed for a natural home birth. Not only did we apply our faith, but we applied our actions. We read all the books! We watched all the videos. We enrolled in the classes.

I shifted the blame from God, and I started blaming myself. I felt as though our admission to the hospital was an unanswered prayer because of something I may have done. I began searching my life for the past nine months for things that I may have done to offend God. When I couldn't find anything, I told myself that I must have misinterpreted or disobeyed God's voice somewhere along Tianka's pregnancy journey. And so, I dug deeper inside my past to figure out where I went wrong. I felt like an absolute failure! I questioned my faith; I second-guessed my relationship with God. I asked myself, "*Do you really know God?*"

"*Have I been receptible of his voice?*"

When I had no more words left to humiliate myself before God and to dispute with God, that's when the Holy Spirit reminded me of the story of Job, the perfect man who did everything right, yet, he lost everything. The Holy Spirit said to me, "Just because you did everything right doesn't mean that you will be exempted from trials, tests or that your prayers will be answered." "It is the Father's will that prevails over your desires." The Holy Spirit began to minister to my distraught soul. He reminded me about the life of Jesus, the Son of God, who conquered sin by living a perfect life by doing everything right. Yet, He had to experience the one thing that He prayed three times for His Father to exempt him from the burden of the cross. This brought peace to my soul.

I washed my face and waited until the redness of my eyes were clear. I returned to the room as though nothing was wrong with me. I had on my game face. By the time I had gotten to the room, the Pitocin that was ordered came, and they were ready to administer it. Seeing Tianka hooked up with so many tubes was daunting for me. Nothing in that hospital room looked like anything that we had prayed, planned, imagined, or hope would happen.

I remember looking in Tianka's eyes and seeing the confidence that she had in me trapped inside her eyes. I held her hands, and I told her that she had been doing an awesome job and that everything was going to be fine. She said, "Okay baby," and tears started rolling down my eyes once more. Again, I just felt like I was responsible for her being in the hospital because I might have misinterpreted God's voice. Tears started rolling down her eyes just the same.

Emergency C-section

As the night progressed, Tianka received a higher dosage of Pitocin. After the final dosage, they realized that the baby wasn't responding well to the higher dosage of Pitocin. Our baby's heart rate began to fluctuate. By this time, it was around 5:30am on Monday, June 18, 2018, Tianka's doctor came back to do a check-up. He checked her cervix and unfortunately, it still hadn't dilated any further. We knew what was coming next. He explained that her cervix was unchanged and that the baby wasn't coping well with the increased dosage of Pitocin. He said that there wasn't another way to proceed without risking the baby going into sudden distress. We asked how soon she had to undergo the c-section, and his response was, "Now!." He left the room and gave us five minutes to make a decision.

Suddenly, Tianka broke down! I felt helpless. Her mom, who had done two c-sections was on a video call via Skype, and so she encouraged her and talked her through the process. Her aunt also encouraged her. We prayed and then welcomed back the nurse in the room to prepare Tianka for surgery.

A Sudden Peace

*"I am leaving you with a gift—peace of mind and heart. And the peace I give is a gift the world cannot give. So don't be troubled or afraid. - **John 14:27 (NLT)***

Before labor, my wife was never mentally prepared to have a c-section. Therefore, I was surprised at the sudden peace, calmness, courage, and strength that my wife displayed. It's almost as if once she realized what was needed to be done, she adjusted. As for me, I was never prepared to walk into an actual surgical room to support my wife through a c-section. I was already having difficulties watching surgeries being performed in televised medical drama series such a Greys Anatomy. I typically get light-headed at the sight of excessive blood. However, as soon as I stepped into that surgical room, I felt like a wave of divine peace hit me. I was able to maintain internal and external composure, and this time, it wasn't fake. Without a shadow of a doubt, we met God in that surgical room.

During her procedure, she felt nauseated and intoxicated by the drugs. She didn't want to feel any pain, so that was working to her advantage. However, what the doctors never told her was that even though she took an epidural, she was going to feel intense pressure. While the doctors were pulling the baby out, she screamed! She mentioned that at one point, everything became blurry, and she began heading towards a pink light. However, she was able to convince herself to snap out of it. As the doctors pulled her baby out, she described the sensation as though a 12,000-pound elephant was sitting on top of her. Again, she screamed! She asked the doctor to slow down. He said, "Sure," but pulled the baby out suddenly. She made her final scream! After an hour-long surgery, Geor'nyah Eliana Morrison, meaning God's gift to us, was born on Monday, June 18, 2018, at 6:30 am. Everything vanished once Tianka heard the sound of her baby's voice. After seeing and touching her baby, her heart was full.

The baby and I were at one side of the operation room, where they administered various tests and measurements. After about 30 minutes, Tianka got to hold her baby. She was marveled at the beauty of her little one. Our support team later joined us in the recovery room. After an hour, we were all moved to the postnatal ward where Tianka and the baby received further care.

Later on, a nurse came in and told us that depending on Tianka and the baby's health, we could leave the hospital in only a matter of 3-4 days. We knew it was only a possibility, however after the entire experience that we've been through and how restless we've been for the past couple of days, we needed something to look forward to, and that was going home. Therefore, we had high hopes that we were going home soon enough.

Emergency Neonatal Intensive Care Unit (NICU) Admission

At around 2:30 am on Tuesday, June 19, 2018, a nurse awakened Tianka and me. She told us that she needed our baby for basic newborn screening. I went with them and waited as they performed several tests. The waiting area was freezing, so I told the nurse I was heading back to our room. I asked her to inform me once she's finished. I fell asleep, but although I was sleeping, I was subconsciously awaiting the nurse's call. Hours had passed, and she didn't call. I didn't think anything of it, so I continued sleeping. At around 6 a.m, a nurse from the neonatal intensive care unit came and told us that our baby was urgently admitted. He explained that Geor'nyah had low oxygen in her blood; therefore, her heart had an irregular beat. He stated that they weren't sure if it was associated with a lung or heart defect. Therefore, she was admitted for further observation. He mentioned that a cardiologist was going to examine her to determine if she has critical congenital heart disease (CCHD).

Although the challenges that Tianka encountered may be trivial matters to what some mothers have experienced during childbirth, I must say it was still hard for her. And yes, there are also mothers whose child has battled with illnesses more severe than what our child had to contend. However, it's still frightening to hear that your child is admitted. As first time parents, the news hit us pretty hard. We never imagined our baby being admitted as a result of health defects. It felt as if every time we thought the storm was over and that there was going to be peace and safety, something disruptive was on the verge of happening.

We went to visit our baby girl. It was difficult to see her hooked up to an oxygen tank, cardiopulmonary monitor, and a bunch of other machines. She looked so fragile. The doctors explained that she was going to be admitted for a while. Tianka was so disheartened.

A day had passed, and after several blood tests, a nurse informed us that our baby didn't have critical congenital heart disease CCHD. He explained that she had birth asphyxia. This is a condition that occurs when a newborn's brain or organs isn't receiving adequate oxygen. In her case, her heart wasn't receiving sufficient oxygen. They placed her on a breathing support machine until she could breathe properly on her own. Seeing her going from one extreme to another was heartbreaking. I can only imagine how tiresome this whole process might have been for her.

Two days later, the doctors cleared Tianka for home. We were advised that we had to check out of our room. The only issue was, our baby was still admitted to the NICU, and she was going to be there for an additional three to four days. Tianka was also breastfeeding every three hours per day. She was adamant about not using baby formula despite the immense pressure that we received from a few of the NICU nurses to give her baby formula. When Tianka refused to submit to the nurses' suggestion, it caused some opposition. A few of the nurses who were responsible for monitoring our baby disliked her. They occasionally made smart disrespectful comments, and their body language was always negative towards her.

Tianka wasn't just going to roll over and play dead. She wasn't going to go home and leave our baby at the mercy of those nurses. We prayed, asking God to provide a way. After praying, the Spirit led us to speak to the manager of the postnatal ward. To our amusement, she allowed us to stay free of charge until our baby was released. Staying also meant that Tianka would no longer receive any medical care from any of the nurses unless she was re-admitted.

We weren't fully prepared for the long week that was ahead of us. We needed more clothes and such. And being that our baby slept for three hours after being fed, we had a three-hour window to rush back home and grab some stuff.

Chapter Six

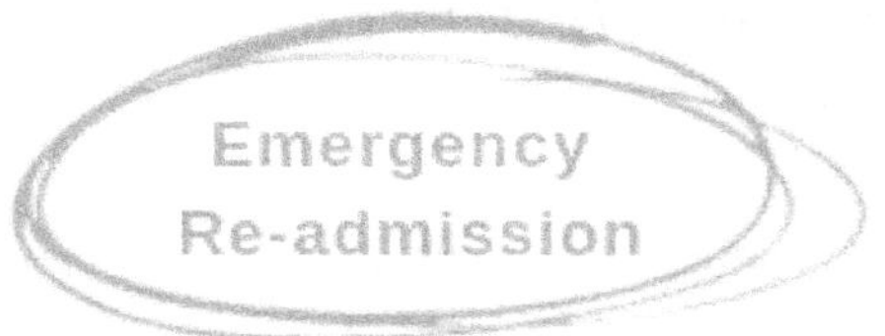

At around 12:00 am on Thursday, June 21, 2018, Tianka was re-admitted to the emergency room. She kept having chills. She would get extremely cold or hot. Given that she was released from the hospital's care, she started to monitor and record the timing of her pain killer medication intake as well as her temperature. All seemed fine with her temperature except for when she would get the chills or hot flashes an hour or so before she took her medication. She thought nothing of it since after taking her medication, her temperature would be fine, plus she was more focused on resting and getting to the NICU to feed the baby every three hours.

A nurse that was fond of us came to check on Tianka although she was discharged. She checked Tianka's temperature and thought it was a little high, however,

Tianka's doctor said it was fine since her temperature didn't remain high (due to her taking the medication).

The Thursday evening, of June 21, our church friends (Agatha & Nadra) came to visit. They brought us food and was checking in with Tianka's general progress. Tianka mentioned the fever situation, and they suggested that she should stop taking the medication and monitor her true temperature. After they left, Tianka stopped taking the medication and began to monitor her temperature. At around 11 pm, Tianka began to feel extremely cold. Cold sweat was stomping out of her pores. I checked her temperature, and it was 103.4. Although she was discharged, she called the nurses station, but they disregarded us. When a nurse decided to answer our phone call, we were told that Tianka was discharged and was no longer under the care of the hospital. Therefore, they are unable to help us in any way. Although they were right, and it was just the hospital's policy, it was disheartening to see how insensitive people or organizational rules can be. Another nurse told us that Tianka was likely having a fever because her milk supply was coming in and that we shouldn't be too concerned. She didn't even take the time to check Tianka's body temperature. I knew she didn't care and that she was saying that to dismiss us.

Without hesitating, we called Tianka's aunt as well as Nadra, and they both advised me to take Tianka to the emergency room.

Once in the emergency room, Tianka immediately explained what was happening. Once she gave them the record of her temperature, and the nature of her birth, everything started to move fast again.

Suddenly, Tianka was rushed to a room where two nurses began to withdraw blood and pump fluid. Shortly after another nurse came to administer a chest x-ray, and it seemed as if for three-four hours straight, Tianka was being tested and retested for post-op infections.

The result showed that Tianka had developed an infection as a result of the meconium (baby poop) that was released inside of her body before delivery. They also suspected that the infection was also influenced by the fact that her membrane was ruptured for so long.

She was immediately treated with antibiotics.

Our baby was still admitted to the NICU, and we both were still being pressured to give her baby formula. What was ironic about this situation was that the walls of the NICU were plastered with posters encouraging moms to breastfeed.

Despite the antibiotics that Tianka was taking, the doctors gave Tianka the green light to breastfeed. That was good news for her! Regardless of how ill and tired Tianka was, she was still pumping breast milk, and I was taking them to the nurses at the NICU so they could feed our baby. Now and then, I would check up on our baby to see how she was doing. I can still remember the sound of her heart monitor, her yellow eyes that peeped at me, and the overwhelming aroma of antibiotics that stained her body and clothing. I would speak to the nurses about her progress and then head back to support Tianka.

I informed our church community that Tianka was re-admitted, and in the blink of an eye, our friends (Agatha and Nadra) were back at the hospital. They brought us more food and stayed in support of Tianka and the baby. We talked, joked, and prayed.

We stayed at the hospital for an additional three days. On the third day, we got word from Tianka and our baby girl's doctors that they were stabilized enough to leave, we were so ecstatic!

Your Story

Dear mother,

Congratulations on the conception of your child. Children are truly a gift from the Lord, and they are a reward from him. - *Psalm 127:3* (NLT)

My wife's c-section was life-changing because of all the lessons that we both learned.

Here are a few of the most important lessons that Tianka learned:

1. Always be Thankful - I prayed many years for a child. After every negative pregnancy test, I would cry tears of frustration for many nights. Finally, I conceived. I prayed, hoped, and believed for natural unmedicated childbirth. However, that was not my reality.

    My daughter's birth taught me to be still in the process and to always be thankful for answered prayers regardless of how they manifest themself. For me, I am overjoyed to have had the birth I did and everything that came with it as opposed to not being pregnant at all. In all things, always give thanks. Lord, I thank you from the bottom of my heart for our baby girl; she is truly a blessing.

2. Don't Allow Fear to Cripple your Joy - I feared having a C-section, so when labor wasn't progressing, I started to become crippled by the fact that I would have to undergo a C-section. That fear took away the joy of living in the moment and calmly breathing through each contraction and enjoying the beauty of labor. It also made me feel incompetent as a mother because my body was unable to do what it was meant to do.

   Whenever I'm faced with a situation that can rob me of my joy, and the opportunity to see the beauty in my situation. I remind myself to calmly breathe and to know that it's going to be okay. '

   My sincere prayer is that you'll have a safe childbirth and one that you desire. However, if your childbirth isn't going the way you planned, know that it's natural to feel fearful, however, take a deep breath, know that you and your baby are going to be okay and do your best to not allow that fear to consume you. Enjoy the beauty of your childbirth.

3. Always have a "Plan B"- Having a "Plan B" or even a "plan C" doesn't mean you dont have faith or confidence in "Plan A. Having alternate plans to your

ideal childbirth and being okay with those plans will make you more comfortable and calm in the event you have to switch to them.

Now, whenever I'm planning my life, I leave an open mind and room on my notepad to write my "Plan B or C."

Here are a few of the most important lessons that I learned:

1. Gratefulness – As I laid on the small couch in our hospital room, and looked through the window that overlooked the city, I felt angry at God and at life for the childbirth experience that both Tianka and I encountered. I was so exhausted that I felt like it robbed me of the excitement and joy that I was supposed to feel after the birth of our daughter on Father's Day. Then the Holy Spirit led me to my Facebook page, and one of my high school mates posted this message " I didn't get to be a father very long, but I feel GRATEFUL and blessed for the 17 hours that I was."

Through my school mate's message, God showed me how ungrateful I was and that regardless of what I'm going through, somebody else is going through worst. I dragged myself out of self-pity, praised God for His wonderful blessing, and changed my attitude. To this day, I rejoice, and I'm forever grateful for everything that happens in my life.

2. Selfless Love – Imagine yourself spending nine (9) months to establish a plan that's stacked with your desires. Now imagine being in a situation where you must surrender all of your wants, boundaries, and desires within that plan in less than twenty-four hours for someone you love. *Do you think you could be selfless that quick?*

When I saw my wife being sliced open on that surgery table on the morning of June 18, 2018, I also saw all of her desires and preferences from her pregnancy plan being sliced.

She never wanted to do a c-section; she never wanted to have an epidural, pitocin, or any of the drugs that were given to her for pain relief. To see her cry through it and put her baby's life above her health and preferences taught me what it truly meant to love someone selflessly. Selfless love requires great sacrifice. Today, in all that I do for my wife and child, I do it selflessly.

3. Respect - Like most other mothers, Tianka had a rough pregnancy and childbirth experience. Bearing witness to it allowed me to develop a deeper sense of admiration for her womanly strength and character. Above all, it taught me how to honor her in my words and actions.

4. Bond – Whether Tianka had a C-section or not, her giving birth to my child would have been enough to strengthen our bond. However, her having a c-section has further tightened the knot in our marriage and has allowed us to develop a stronger emotional connection with each other.

Throughout your nine months journey, you will be exposed to the birth stories of others through strangers, friends, family, videos, social media, or doctors. Some of these stories will be encouraging & some will discourage you. Above all, remember that labor & delivery is unpredictable & no number of stories can truly determine how your birth story will end. Your story will be unique. Your only true way of discovering which method of delivery is suitable for your baby and your body is to experience childbirth itself.

A natural birth, a medicated birth or a surgical birth is only considered to be bad if it results in any life-long effect or a fatal outcome of the baby, mom, or both. If the baby or mother makes it outside the hospital walls in a healthy condition from either one of these delivery methods, then you've just experienced a safe & supernatural birth.

Regardless of which birthing method you experience, be grateful, and be blessed with your own birth story.

God is with you!

Chapter Seven

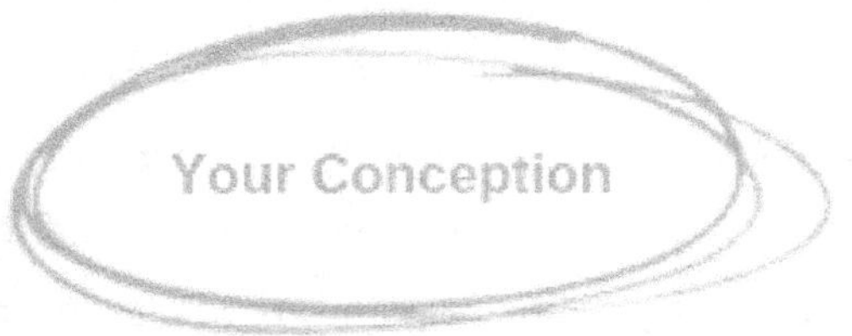

Your conception is a beautiful blessing that's about to add a brand new meaning to your life. It's a true depiction of God's perfect timing and favor. If you conceived your child through non-consensual intercourse, then God personally told me to tell you that your child is a gift given from Heaven and not from the perpetrator. Therefore, release yourself from the shackles of guilt, shame, and possibly self-blame. The life inside your womb is about to take you on one of life's most rewarding journey. To all pregnant moms, you are beautiful, you are strong, you are fearless, and you got this!

You may have conceived at a time in your life when it seems like you may not have all the right resources.

However, know that you and your baby are a child of God, and God knows the exact need of His children before they even realize that they have a need. And like a good Father, He only gives His children good gifts. (See *Matthew 6:8 & Luke 11:13*) Therefore, don't be afraid to laugh, dance, or cry tears of joy over the newly discovered fetus that will bring you, or you and your family tremendous joy, and favor. Celebrate your moment! If you haven't revealed the good news to your partner, or your family or friends, then plan a private or public pregnancy reveal to inform them.

Chapter Eight

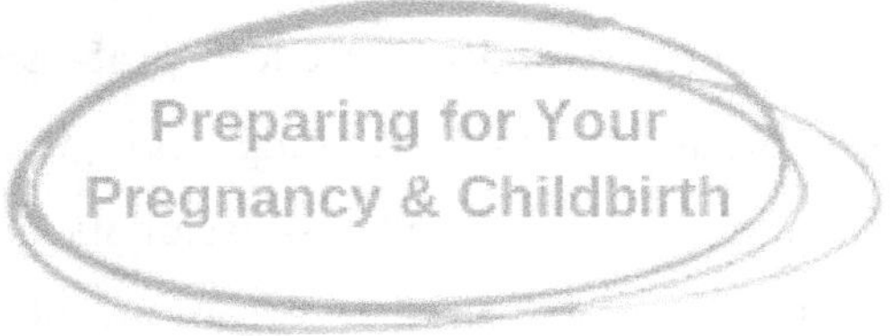

Preparation involves gathering resources and doing the necessary research to make available the best possible measures for the next nine months of you and your baby's life. Here are some key things that you should know that will ensure that you're prepared for childbirth.

Education

My people are destroyed for lack of knowledge.
- Hosea 4:6 (KJV)

Education is the golden rule for success in any new endeavor. Through educating yourself, you'll attain the necessary information, resources, and professionalism that will help you make informed decisions that will lead to success. When it comes to childbirth, educating yourself about pregnancy and childbirth is the golden rule that will help you make informed decisions throughout your pregnancy and childbirth. You can educate yourself about pregnancy and childbirth through reading books, reading blog articles from certified and trusted professionals or health-care organizations, watching pregnancy and childbirth videos from certified professionals or health-care organizations on youtube, and from attending birth classes.

When You Should See A Doctor

Once you've found out that you're pregnant, you may have a lot of questions going through your mind. One of them may be, "*When should I see a doctor?* " That's a great question. As soon as you suspect that you're pregnant, you are required to schedule an appointment with a health-care provider such as an obstetrician/gynecologist. If you've confirmed your pregnancy with a home pregnancy test, it's still wise to follow-up with a doctor's appointment. This will ensure that you and your baby are off to a great start.

Choosing the Right Primary Health-Care Provider

Pregnancy, as well as labor and delivery, will be one of the most vulnerable points of your life. Therefore, who your prenatal care provider will be is a sensitive and personal matter. In many cases and for various reasons, the health care provider that did your first pre-natal consultation may not be the health care provider that you want to remain with throughout your pregnancy. Therefore, this is where selecting the right health-care provider becomes another important factor to consider. Having a health-care provider that can offer their professional service of monitoring your pregnancy or help you deliver a bouncing baby is great. However, because most mothers are typically emotionally vulnerable during the stages of pregnancy, labor, and delivery, especially when unforeseen complications arise. You'll need a health-care provider that has a level of empathy to step outside of their professional acumen when needed, to help you get through those rocky stages. Also, it's important to know that whoever you select as your health-care provider, whether it's an obstetrician or a midwife, please ensure that you fish out their character to determine if they possess some or all of the qualities I will list below. If they don't, then you may want to consider someone else as your health-care provider.

Emotional Quotient

Emotional quotient (intelligence) is a person's ability to identify, manage, and steer their own emotions as well as the emotions of others in a positive direction, especially in challenging moments. Currently, in certain industries, a person's level of emotional intelligence is used to determine if he or she is qualified for a job. It's done by taking an emotional test. The theory is that someone with high emotional intelligence would make a better leader because they can connect with people by steering their negative emotions or thoughts about themselves or a situation in a positive direction for them to overcome a challenge or to accomplish a task.

When it comes to pregnancy and emotions, studies have shown that the production of hormones such as progesterone and estrogen is likely to increase throughout a woman's pregnancy. This hormonal increase is known to have an impact on your emotions, thus making you more emotional than usual. In fact, you may experience high surges of irritability, sadness, tearfulness, anxiety, or depression. Likewise, labor and delivery can also be filled with such outbursts of emotions ranging from irritability, sadness, tearfulness, anxiety, or depression for new moms. They commonly experience a flood of negative emotions and thoughts when things aren't going according to their birth plan. In moments like these, you'll need a health-care provider that's able to understand what you're going through and able connect with you emotionally when needed at different stages of your pregnancy as well as labor and delivery.

Tianka had many challenges to overcome throughout her pregnancy and labor. Many of which had her on an emotional rollercoaster ride. At times she was experiencing emotions that she couldn't articulate. And when labor wasn't going according to Tianka's birth plan, she felt anxious, sad, tearful, and depressed. In these moments, her midwife could not identify, label, and differentiate both her and Tianka's emotions. She also could not conceal her fearful and doubtful emotions. They were always portrayed through her responses, words, and body language. In every moment that seemed to produce a sinister outcome, our midwife freaked out. That had a domino effect on us. When Tianka was about to be transferred to the hospital, our midwife was so overwhelmed by negative emotions that she didn't even fill out the application form correctly. We had to fill out a new application form the moment we got to the hospital. The funny thing is that our midwife is a certified professional. But, she wasn't certified enough to identify and maneuver Tianka's emotions or thoughts in a positive direction despite the many setbacks. I am not saying that you should attempt to put your potential health-care provider through a rigorous emotional intelligence test. However, there are subtle ways of screening your health-care provider to determine if he or she is the right fit.

Here are a few signs of an emotionally intelligent professional can be used to help you choose the right primary health-care provider for you and your baby:

- **They're Patient –** When you go in for your prenatal care visit(s), *does your health-care provider listens to your pregnancy updates, concerns, or your challenges without showing any signs of annoyance? Is your health-care provider patient while answering your questions, or does he or she always seems annoyed when you ask questions? Does your health-care provider allow you to finish your complaints or questions without forcing you to cut it short so they can move onto the next patient? Does he or she fidget while you're expressing your complaints, questions, or concerns?* Signs of impatience are often expressed in restless body languages such as the tapping of feet or fingers, constantly shifting in their chairs, doodling, or even checking a Smartphone.

Pregnancy is a very delicate time in a woman's life. It's a time when you are most vulnerable and sensitive to the things (words, actions, or body language) that you encounter daily. Therefore, you're going to be concerned about finding answers to the constant changes that are taking place within your body. Finding a health-care provider that can accommodate your questions and concerns, and that can articulate his or her answers clearly and concisely is a quality that's not worth a compromise. If your health-care provider is annoyed and impatient with you during the easiest stage of your pregnancy, then chances are he or she will be impatient and sometimes annoyed with you throughout the hardest stages— pregnancy complications, labor, and delivery.

During early labor, Tianka had a lot of questions and concerns; however, her midwife was incapable of properly articulating what was happening to her. All of her answers were abrupt. Her body language and smart comments made it clear that we were asking too many questions. However, after Tianka was transferred under the hospital's care, the nurses answered her questions, even before she asked them. They were also patient, and they listened well.

- **They're Empathetic** – When explaining your thoughts, feelings, or condition; was your health-care provider able to understand your thoughts, feelings, or condition from your perspective, rather than his or her point of view? Did he or she express compassion when your situation or condition required it?

  I'm not advising you to be overly demanding of empathic behavior from your health-care provider because it is believed that too much empathy interferes with rational decision making. However, your health-care provider must be able to strike a balance between applying their professional expertise to solve a problem and applying empathy to connect with a person to promote optimism and help the person accomplish a task.

- **They're good listeners** – During consultations or prenatal visits, do you feel like you have to compete for your health-care provider's attention? Do you always have to repeat yourself during your prenatal visit? Can he or she summarize what you've just told them? If your health-care provider can't summarize what you've shared and let you know what they suspect to be the cause of your condition, then there's a possibility that he or she hasn't been listening to you. Sometimes they may even ask you to go back to square one. Does he or she request you to do unnecessary tests?

- **They show authenticity** – Does your health-care provider follow up on your symptoms, questions, or concerns? Does he or she have a sincere desire to understand and consider your best interest, symptoms, questions, or concerns? Does he or she treat your questions, concerns, symptoms, or your explanations with a level of importance or urgency?

  Does he or she go the extra mile to ensure that you understand something? Does he or she make your prenatal visits a priority?

  When your health-care provider can display a level of care and sincerity for you and your baby's health despite the pressure of so many daily tasks staring at them, it shows that they'll be able to effectively care for you throughout the stress and unpredictable challenges of pregnancy, labor, and delivery.

- **They give helpful feedback** – When there are challenges with your health or your baby's health, *does your health-care provider always respond with negative feedback?* Whenever Tianka was battling with health issues during her pregnancy, her midwife's response always sounded critical and harsh. When it came to labor, she demonstrated the same negative response to every arising challenge. At times it was clear that she was talking down at us.

- When it comes to your pregnancy and childbirth, you'll need helpful feedback. If you detect that your health-care provider lacks these attributes or any other attribute that's not compromisable for you, then it is best to steer clear.

Choosing a Secondary Health-Care Provider

Having a back-up doctor is like packing extra clothing and shoes for your girl's trip in case of any unforeseen situation.

In case your primary health-care provider is unable to assist you throughout the entire duration of your pregnancy, or childbirth, having a secondary health-care provider allows you to transition and receive medical attention and care that you and your baby need.

When Tianka's primary health-care provider was unable to further assist with childbirth, Tianka's secondary health-care provider filled in perfectly. Also, always check-in with your primary health-care provider to ensure that he or she is updating your secondary health-care provider with information about your pregnancy from your first to your final trimester. You must also occasionally check-in with your secondary health-care provider to ensure he or she is receiving your pregnancy updates.

Nutrition

" Whatever you eat, your baby eats, and whatever your baby eats will determine his or her health.

Throughout your pregnancy, you must give your child the best start at life by taking careful consideration of the food, beverage, or medication that you'll consume during pregnancy. You do this by becoming intentional about the medication, food, or beverage that you'll consume by reading the labels that are found on products and researching the ingredients so that you're aware of the harmful ingredients to avoid. You also create a meal plan based on your research and getting insight from your health-care provider or a dietitian. Doing this allows you to make informed choices about the food or beverage that you'll be consuming.

Here are a few foods and ingredients to avoid:

- **Fish with mercury** - Fish that are high in mercury are known to hinder brain development and cause brain damage. Some of these fishes are king mackerel, shark, swordfish, etc.

  Solution: You may eat fish such as salmon, catfish, cod, and canned light tuna, all of which are rich in omega-3 fatty acids and low in mercury. The high protein, low saturated fats, and many essential nutrients contribute to the child's heart and brain development.

- **Raw shellfish** - Raw shellfish such as oysters, clams, and mussels contain harmful bacteria, viruses, and toxins that will cause seafood-borne illnesses. Therefore, it's recommended that you avoid these throughout your pregnancy.

- **Solution:** Instead of eating raw shellfish, you can eat cooked shellfish. Ensure that you cook them with their shells open.

- **Raw meat and poultry** - Eating raw, rare or undercooked meats are highly dangerous as it contains a harmful parasite called Toxoplasma and a harmful bacteria called Salmonella. Toxoplasma causes toxoplasmosis that results in flu-like symptoms, which develop a few weeks after consumption of the food. It can lead to miscarriage or fetal death during delivery, while salmonella increases the risk of food poisoning.

Solution: You must eat well-cooked meat at the correct temperature.

- **Deli meats –** Deli meats are also known as cold cuts, luncheon meats, cooked meats, sliced meats, or cold meats. These types of meats are often precooked or cured and served cold. They are often sausages or meatloaves. They are known to contain listeria bacteria, which can readily move from the mother to the placenta, causing severe complications, including fetal death.

Solution: Cooking at a high temperature is known to kill listeria. Therefore, you should eat deli meats after reheating or as a meal served hot.

- **Raw or undercooked eggs** - Raw, undercooked, or soft-boiled eggs should be avoided as they also contain harmful salmonella bacteria. The salmonella bacteria cause food poisoning. Once a pregnant mother has contracted the salmonella bacteria, they may experience diarrhea, severe vomiting, headache, abdominal pain, and high temperature. These symptoms are unlikely to harm a mother's baby;

however, it weakens a mother's immune system. Ultimately, this affects the baby's development. Also, foods that contain raw eggs such as homemade Caesar dressings, custards, ice creams, mayonnaise, Béarnaise sauce, Aioli sauce, and desserts, including mousse, tiramisu, and meringue must be avoided.

Solution: Eat cooked eggs that contain firm yolks or well-cooked omelets, and salads. Also, purchase pasteurized egg products as pasteurization will reduce the risk of food-borne illness in dishes that are not cooked or are lightly cooked.

- **Unwashed fruits and vegetables** – When fruits & vegetables are left unwashed, you run the risk of consuming harmful pathogens such as Toxoplasma parasite. The Toxoplasma parasite can cause serious complications in babies, such as vision and learning problems.

Solution: Rinse the fruits and vegetables thoroughly with a vegetable wash. Also, peel away or scrub the surfaces and cut off the bruised areas, as they are prone to bacteria.

- **Excess caffeine** - Caffeine can be found in tea, chocolate, and energy drinks. Some research reveals that excessive caffeine intake is associated with premature birth and withdrawal symptoms in infants. Some studies also state that it increases a mother's chances of miscarriage. Therefore, pregnant moms should limit caffeine intake to less than 200 mg per day.

Solution: Opt for decaffeinated beverages, especially in your first trimester, as the risk of miscarriage is high.

- **Canned foods** – Almost all canned food contains an epoxy liner containing Bisphenol A (BPA), this is a toxic substance that affects the fetal endocrine activity and causes fertility problems, cancer, liver ailments, and heart diseases in pregnant women. They are thought to cause reproductive issues, slow brain development, and behavioral problems in children. In most cases, they harbor harmful bacteria due to their long shelf life.

Solution: Avoid canned foods altogether.

- **Artificial Nitrate** – Artificial nitrate is a preservative that is used to enhance a food's color and to improve its shelf life. Nitrate can be found in foods such as cured sandwich meats, bacon, salami, or sausages to give them their pink, reddish color and to prolong their shelf life. Upon consumption, nitrates turn to nitrosamines in the body, increasing the chances of cancer molecules in mothers, and abnormalities in the fetus.

Solution: Avoid eating these foods that are rich in nitrate.

And remember, during your pregnancy, you must be intentional about giving your baby the best chance of living a healthy life. You'll achieve this by researching about the food, as well as its ingredients before consumption.

The Importance of Taking Prenatal Vitamins

A fetus requires certain nutrients for healthy growth and brain development. Therefore taking a right prenatal vitamin throughout the entire duration of your pregnancy is paramount to having a healthy baby and an intelligent child. These types of nutrients are compacted in a capsule that is called prenatal vitamins. If your meal plan for the duration of your pregnancy is exempted from certain key food groups, then taking prenatal vitamins is the perfect way to bridge the gap and optimize your meal plan.

How to Know Which Prenatal Vitamin is Right for You

When searching for a prenatal vitamin that's right for you, here is a list of the most important ingredients that make up a good prenatal vitamin supplement:

- **Folic acid -** Folic acid is a special type of B complex vitamin that's found in green vegetables, kidney, and liver. Taking folic acid before and during pregnancy helps your body to create that extra blood that you need during pregnancy. It's also known to help prevent congenital disabilities of your baby's brain and spinal cord. Doctor's findings have shown that most congenital disabilities occur within the first two-three weeks of pregnancy. Therefore, it's paramount that you have folic acid in your system during those early stages of your pregnancy when your baby's brain and spinal cord are developing.

- **Calcium -** Calcium is an essential mineral for all pregnant women and their babies. Having a proper calcium intake will help your baby or babies to develop strong, healthy teeth, bones, heart, muscles, and nerves. Studies have also shown that a high calcium diet increases your baby's chance of being born with a normal heart rhythm. Also, proper calcium intake is known to fortify mom's breast milk.

- **Vitamin D** - This vitamin is an essential mineral that is known to help both mom and baby absorb calcium. Getting ample vitamin D is also known to prevent a skeletal disorder known as rickets disease, which can lead to abnormal bone growth, deformity, fracture, delayed, or faulty physical development.

- **Iron** - During pregnancy, a mother's body works overtime; therefore, it requires twice the amount of nutritional supplements to keep mom and the baby healthy. When it comes to iron, a mother needs twice the amount of iron to produce that extra blood that her body desperately needs to ensure that herself and her baby's organs and cells have the adequate blood supply to receive oxygen.

Based on your medical history and your current medical record, you may consult with your health-care provider or a dietician to find out which prenatal vitamins are right for you and the dosage that you'll need. I have included a few natural, high-quality prenatal vitamins that every mom should take in the resource section of this book.

The Importance of Having a Birth Plan

During childbirth, things have a way of shifting course swiftly. It's easy to get carried away in those moments, having a birth plan present during childbirth reduces the risk of you being left uninformed of doctor's/midwife's decisions in the spur of the moment. Your birth plan is a document that will outline detailed information about the things that you desire to occur or not to happen throughout childbirth. It will be one of your strongest communicators to articulate your desires. Having a birth plan also allows your health-care provider and everyone else who will be a part of your childbirth support team about the type of childbirth you'd like to have.

Important Things to Include in Your Birth Plan

There are myriad of things to consider when formulating a birth plan. Here are a few essentials to include in your birth:

- **Method of delivery** - When you think about delivery methods, you think about how you would want your baby to be delivered. Do you want a natural hospital childbirth? Do you want a natural home birth? Do you want a medicated childbirth? Do you want to have a planned c-section? Do you want to have a vaginal birth after c-section (VBAC)? These are all the different methods of childbirth that must be considered. Our advice is that you consider two outcomes. These two outcomes are:

Your best possible outcome - The best possible outcome for most pregnant women is to have a natural vaginal birth where they get to experience the natural sensation of childbirth without medical intervention.

Your worst possible outcome - The worst possible outcome for most pregnant women is to prepare for a natural birth only to experience a hospital birth or an emergency c-section. Therefore, they make secondary preparations for another method of childbirth in case of unforeseen complications.

From the two outcomes, it's highly recommended that every mom chooses a method of delivery as her best and worst outcome. You should pray, prepare, and hope to experience your best possible outcome. However, you must also pray, prepare, and hope to overcome your worst possible outcome in case it becomes your reality.

Pain Relief Methods

The pain relief method that you choose will be dependent on your method of childbirth. When you think about having a medicated birth, you think about taking nitrous oxide, pethidine, or the most common drug of them all—epidural anesthesia. When you think about experiencing natural childbirth, you think about including non-medical techniques such as massages, essential oils, music, hot or cold packs, warm shower, immersion in a warm bath, and the most important one of them all—proper breathing technique. Whichever childbirth method you chose, you must research and educate yourself about the various pain relief methods and their side effects.

Here's a brief insight into the most common medical pain relief methods, and their side effects:

- **Nitrous oxide** - Nitrous oxide is also known as "Laughing gas." When your anxiety gets in the way of childbirth, nitrous oxide is a gas that'll be provided through a mask. You'll be required to inhale the gas as needed. Once inhaled, it doesn't guarantee an escape from pain; however, it will calm your tense nerves and cause you to relax. The side effects of nitrous oxide are headaches, shivering, excessive sweating, nausea, vomiting, and fatigue.

- **Pethidine** – Is a strong pain reliever that is kin to the narcotic family of morphine and heroin. It works by reducing the sensation of pain. It causes you to relax, and it makes you feel sleepy. If required, your health-care provider will inject the pethidine into your thigh. The side effects of Pethidine are: It makes you feel sick; therefore, it will be given along with another drug that's called an anti-emetic. Anti-emetic is used to control nausea and vomiting. Pethidine also slows down your breathing. Therefore, you'll need oxygen through a face mask. This drug will also make your baby drowsy for several days after birth. It is also proven to affect the placenta and may affect your baby's breathing.

- **Epidural anesthesia** – This is the most dominant and most effective pain relief for childbirth. If required, epidural anesthesia will be injected into the epidural space around the spinal cord. The substance is then passed through a thin tube that will be installed to your back. Epidural anesthesia will numb your belly and the lower portion of your body. Unlike other drugs, it allows you to stay awake and to be alert during vaginal or c-section childbirth. During a c-section, you won't feel any pain when the incision is made. However, you are likely to feel an intense pressure when the baby is being pulled out of your stomach. The side effects of an epidural are it can affect your ability to urinate; therefore, you may need a urinary catheter during labor or after your baby's born. It spikes your blood pressure; therefore, you'll be carefully monitored by a nurse. Using epidural also causes constipation. It weakens your leg muscles; therefore, you'll be confined to a bed. You may also experience itchiness, etc.

Overall, none of these pain-relieving drugs completely eradicates, and you will feel pressure or discomfort.

Your Birth Support Team

Childbirth has a way of changing extremes; therefore, you'll need a support team to help you cope through these sudden, unpredictable, and changing circumstances. Tianka and I were blessed to have a self-less support team that was always present with us. We had high hopes for a natural childbirth; however, that dream transitioned to a medicated hospital birth, and then to an emergency c-section. When it came down to deciding if Tianka should do the c-section, our support team helped us in making a solid decision. When fear gripped Tianka, and she needed a release from her fears, her aunt's and mom's words encouraged her to proceed into the operation room confidently.

After our baby was admitted to the NICU (Neonatal intensive care unit) and Tianka was re-admitted to the emergency room, our support team was there to help us. I was restless for four (4) days or more because I had to be there for Tianka and our baby. My body craved for rest, even if it was only for 10 minutes. At that moment, our support team from our church was there to assist Tianka while I slept for an hour.

Regardless of how well you prepare, you never know how your childbirth story will be composed; therefore, you need to ensure that you have adequate help to get you through unforeseen circumstances.

Having the right birth support team is paramount.

Here's a list of things to consider when organizing the right birth team for childbirth:

- **The experienced** - Choosing the right individual means that you'll need to select friends, family members, or a professional that has experience in one of the mentioned childbirth methods (natural birth, hospital birth, c-section, or vaginal birth after c-section). An experienced person will be able to give you solid encouragement and advice that will help you make sound decisions in unforeseen circumstances.

- **The encourager** - You'll need someone who you respect enough that you're willing to receive encouragement from him or her. I'm not saying that you should hire Mr. Les Brown to encourage you through labor and delivery. Having a friend, family member, or a doula that can verbally encourage you through your childbirth will sharpen your countenance to overcome times of fear, doubt, or when you get weary.

- **Intercessor** - The earnest prayer of a righteous person has great power and produces wonderful results. – *James 5: 16 (NLT)*

You'll need someone that knows how to pray, and that can pray for you. Our entire support team was believers. Therefore, we had prayers in abundance, and it produced good results. Tianka didn't experience the type of childbirth that she had planned for; however, both her and our child made it safely out of the hospital despite the many unforeseen challenges.

- **Domestic help** - Having someone on your birth support team that can help you with a variety of light chores can be extremely beneficial! Most of the individuals on our support team were able to cook while I was busy helping Tianka get through labor. Tianka's sister and cousin were able to do minor cleaning, which kept order and a fresh aroma in the environment.

After Tianka was stabilized enough to leave the hospital, we both had to run back home to grab clothes and other stuff. To our realization, the house was a bit messy, our fishes had died, and the house smelled a bit funky. Tianka didn't want to bring the baby home in that environment. She wanted external order in the environment so that she could have internal order and peace when she and the baby got home. It turned out that we had to clean up. At that moment, we wished we had hired someone to get all of our household chores done. Let this be different for you. Get a friend, family member, or hire a cleaner for a few hours to clean your home so that you or your partner don't have to worry about doing it after childbirth. After all, no mother wants to clean a dirty house after experiencing intense pain to bring a child into the world. Besides, the best way to introduce a baby to a new environment is to introduce him or her to a clean environment.

- **Nanny –** If you have more than one child, then hiring a nanny that can solely focus on caring and watching your child or children while you focus on labor and delivery will be very beneficial. Hiring a nanny will also help your birth support team to focus on meeting your needs.

- **General help** - Having someone to hold your hand, wipe your face, give you sips of water, massage your back and shoulders, help you relax, move about, to change position, or to help you with your breathing technique as your contractions intensify will be a sweet medicine for you.

Important Supplies to Include in Your Birth Kit for a Home Birth

- **Your birth plan –** Be sure to issue copies (physical and electronic copies) of your birth plan (both primary & secondary birth plan) to your midwife and every member on your birth support team. Also, be sure to have a copy prepared for your secondary health-care provider in case of a hospital transfer.

- **Birth tub –** If your primary birth plan involves having a home birth, then this means that you'll need to rent or buy a birth tub. Birth tubs can be rented from an independent midwife or a midwife center.

- **Sterile gloves –** If your primary birth plan involves having a home birth, then chances are your midwife will have sterile gloves. However, having a box or a few pairs for back-up purposes won't hurt. Sterile gloves are needed for any examination that your midwife will administer and prevents cross-contamination between health-care providers and patients.

- **Mattress cover, plastic, and clean sheets–** To create a delivery area in your home, cover your mattress with a mattress cover, and then put on a clean sheet. If you're on the floor, have someone help you slide a sheet of plastic (shower curtain) covered with a clean sheet under you.

- **Several dry towels –** After the baby is delivered and placed on mom's bare chest or stomach for skin-to-skin contact, you'll need a towel to dry the baby off. Once the baby is cleaned off: you'll need another dry towel to keep him or her warm.

- **Bulb syringe –** A bulb syringe is a great tool that will be required for usage by your partner, or health-care provider to suction mucus out of your baby's nose to make it easier for he or she to breathe.

- **Isopropyl rubbing alcohol and cotton balls–** This is commonly used to sterilize the scissors that will be used to cut the cord. It can be used to clean your hands, and you can also use it to clean off your baby's umbilical cord along with a cotton ball.

- **Garbage bags –** When your partner is ready to clean the delivery space, with gloves on, roll up the soiled sheets, curtain, and towels, and put them into the bag.

- **Organic coconut water –** Coconut water is known to supply us with all of the five essential electrolytes that our body needs– minerals, sodium, calcium, potassium, and phosphorus. All of these minerals help to soothe the body and provide energy during labor and after childbirth. It also controls blood pressure levels. It also possesses cooling properties, which will cool down your body if you feel hot and sweaty. It also wards off conditions like bilious fever and vomiting.

- **Watermelon Juice –** Like coconut water, watermelon is very hydrating. It has a blast of natural healthy sugars that will give you a kick of energy when you need it the most. Although most health-care providers will forbid you from eating once labor begins, watermelon is perfect for consumption during labor as it's light on the stomach and easy to digest. It's also a perfect after birth snack that will cool you down, keep you hydrated, and restore your energy.

- **Red raspberry leaf herbal tea** – Red raspberry is a plant native to Europe and parts of Asia. It's known for its sweet, nutritious berries and nutrient-packed leaves. Its leaves are used as a herbal tea during labor to strengthen the uterine walls and decrease labor time in a pregnant woman by promoting faster dilation.

- **Organic fruit popsicles** – Although most health-care providers will forbid you from eating once labor begins, other health-care providers believe that eating is fine, especially if it's liquid and if it's light on your stomach. Sucking on a fruit popsicle or two won't cause you any harm. Fruit popsicles are light on the stomach and are known to keep you cool and hydrated during labor. They are packed with vitamins and are known to give you a jolt of energy.

- **Frozen raspberry, blueberry, watermelon or coconut fruit ice cubes** – Fruit Ice cube can be made using raspberry, blueberry, watermelon, coconut water, or your favorite fruit. All you need is a juicer or blender to extract the juice from your fruit, a sieve (strainer) to separate the pulp, a sweetener of your choice (sugar, date, or honey) and an ice cube tray to store the content in your refrigerator. Fruit ice cubes are a quick and easy alternative for fruit popsicles that provides the same cooling effect and nutrients.

- **Snacks (Bananas, grapes, blueberries, nut & seed trail mix)** – In her book – In the Glow What To Eat & Drink During Labor; Carley Mendes states that as labor progresses, a pregnant woman's appetite will naturally decrease as they focus on the task at hand. However, if you're able to eat, then eating small bites of easily digestible snacks such as bananas, grapes, blueberries, nut & seed trail mix contains the necessary vitamins and natural sugars to help you maintain your strength and quench your hunger.

- **Mesh underwear (Postpartum underwear or knit pants)** – Whether you have a vaginal birth or c-section, this underwear is considered to be a lifesaver for a lot of moms. After delivery, these support and recovery underwear will come to your rescue with targeted compression to help reduce swelling and silver-infused fibers that can help eliminate bacteria and odor. They contain leak protection for mothers who bleed heavily after giving birth. For mothers who had a c-section, this underwear doesn't have an elastic waistband that puts pressure on your midsection or the incision line. These are given to you at the hospital, or you can purchase your own.

- **Heating pad** – If you are a fan of a source of warmth, then using a heating pad is a therapeutic way to help you relax sore and tight muscles – especially lower back pain during your pregnancy and labor. If you don't have a heating pad, you can apply a warm blanket to the sore area or take a warm shower.

- **Ice pack –** If you are a fan of a source of coolness, then using an ice pack is also a great therapeutic way to help you relax sore and tight muscles – especially lower back pain during your pregnancy and labor. The choice between a heating pad or an ice pack will be based on your preference and the type of temperature (warm or cool) that your body wants during that moment.

- **Birth ball** – Having a birth ball during your pregnancy and labor will help you to reduce any back pain that you are experiencing. It can also help to ease labor and contraction pain.

- **A playlist with soundtracks, affirmations, instrumentals, or sounds of nature** – Having a playlist with your favorite music can reduce fear and anxiety by helping you to relax. Listening to music provides a positive source of distraction from labor pain. If you're having a hospital birth or giving birth at a midwife center (birth center), then personalizing a playlist is a great way to help make the labor room 'your own' as familiar music will help you to feel in control of your environment.

- **Camera** – For several years now, parent(s) have been able to use a camera to capture one of, if not the most beautiful moments of their life. There's no reason for it to stop now. Having a camera and a photographer (professional or unprofessional) to take pictures of or to video record your special day is a great way to create memories that you can re-live in the future.

With this homebirth checklist, you'll be well prepared for childbirth in the comfort of your home.

Important Supplies to Include in Your Birth Kit for a Hospital Birth

- **Bag or suitcase** – What's a birth kit if you don't have something to store your supplies? Before stacking up on birth supplies, ensure that you have a durable bag or suitcase that's light on the hands, and that can store all of your birth supplies.

- **Your birth plan** – Be sure to issue copies (physical or electronic copies) of your birth plan (both primary &

secondary birth plan) to your health-care provider and every member on your birth support team. Also, be sure to have a copy prepared for your secondary health-care provider in case your primary health-care provider is unable to assist you due to unforeseen circumstances.

- **Toiletries -** A toiletry bag including items such as; Shampoo, conditioner, hairbrush, comb, hair moisturizers, hairdryer, hair clip or band if you have long hair, face soap, face moisturizer, make-up, toothbrush, mouth wash, lip balm, body wash, body lotion, deodorant, and a plastic bag to put dirty clothes in.

- **Clothing** – Breast pads (Helps to stop breast leaks by absorbing the milk), nursing bra (Helps to support swollen, tender breasts, and helps keep breast pads in place.), nightgown or robe (preferably front opening tops for breastfeeding,), both thick and thin socks (If the hospital is cold, thick socks will help keep your feet warm. If the hospital is warm then wearing thin socks will still keep your feet covered and protected without attracting additional warmth to your feet.), slippers, flip flops (to be worn in bathroom or shower.), lots of comfortable underwears, clothing for the trip home,

- **Electronics –** Camera, back-up battery for your camera, memory card (preferably a memory card with a space of 68 -128 gigabytes of space, for video and picture storage) cellphones, cellphone charger,

- **Snacks –** If you aren't eating any snacks during labor, then consider bringing some for your partner and birth support team as well as change for the vending machine.

- **Entertainment –** Like childbirth, the state of your health after giving birth can be unpredictable, which means that your stay at the hospital could be longer than expected. Taking these items will provide some source of entertainment for you, your partner, or the birth support team: books, audiobooks, a tablet, and a Netflix subscription will create the perfect chill vibe.

- **Miscellaneous items –** Some miscellaneous items that will be beneficial are: pillows (Hospital pillows may not be comfortable enough), health insurance card, purse or wallet, partner's driver's license,

With this hospital bag checklist, you'll be well prepared for your time in the hospital.

Important Baby Supplies to Include in Your Birth Kit for a Hospital Birth

- **Baby Bag–** What's a birth kit if you don't have something to store your supplies? Before stacking up on your baby's birth supplies, ensure that you have a durable bag (diaper bag, duffle bag, or baby backpack)that's light on the hands, and that can store all of your baby's birth supplies.

- **Baby clothes-** There's no doubt that you'll receie a few pieces of clothing for your baby, however, packing a few ones, a baby coat or jacket (in case of cold weather) will come in handy.

- **Socks –** Hospitals are usually cold, and newborns tend to get cold easily; therefore, take some baby socks with you.

- **Blankets –** Although hospitals typically provide receiving blankets, taking your own blanket is also good to have for swaddling and coverage during skin to skin contact.

- **Car seat -** While your baby's car seat won't be thrown into your hospital bag, ensure that the right car seat is installed in your car around the same time you pack your baby's bag or as your due date approaches so it's ready for the hospital.

With this baby hospital bag checklist, you'll be well prepared for your time in the hospital.

Important things to Include in Your Birth Kit for Your Birth Support Team

Finally, don't forget about your birth team. Anyone attending the birth, like the father, family member(s), a friend(s), doula, or photographer will need to have substantial food and drink to keep their mood and motivation up while supporting you. You will be better off with foods that don't have a strong smell, which could bother you as labor intensifies.

With this checklist for your birth support team, they will be well prepared for their time to support you at home or at the hospital.

The Importance of Taking a Birth Class

" Childbirth education is an investment that will produce a great return, especially for first-time mothers or parents.

The importance of taking a birth class is that they are loaded with information, practical training, real-life testimonies in real-time, intimate interaction with other mothers, and couples who are anticipating the big day just like you. Another solid reason for signing up for a birth class is that the birth class will contain tips and advice that may not be shared in its entirety by watching YouTube videos or reading blog articles. There are levels to childbirth, and if you aren't fully prepared, then I implore you to reach out to a childbirth educator. As a mom, the more you know about how your body will function during labor, the less fearful you will be about labor and delivery.

Fathers, knowing how your wife's body is going to respond throughout labor and delivery, will help you to prepare mentally, emotionally, and physically for what's ahead. Please, do not approach childbirth from a blind or limited perspective.

Here are a few valuable lessons you will learn in a childbirth class.

Childbirth classes will help you:

- Gain confidence in your body's ability to give birth.

- Gain insight into how to approach a natural, supernatural, medicated, or c-section birth.

- Gain insight into effective and natural pain management strategies.

- Be able to ask questions and talk about your fears with the instructor and other couples.

- It will inform and empower your partner on how to support you throughout your pregnancy and childbirth.

- You'll develop relationships with other moms who have similar pregnancy journey.

- Your partner will gain encouragement and inspiration through interaction with other dads.

- You'll learn about the importance of breastfeeding.

How to Find the Right Birth Class

Here are a few things to consider when searching for a birth class that compliments you or you and your partner's busy schedule:

- **Delivery method -** Selecting the right birth class means that you must register for a childbirth class that's associated with first, your primary delivery method. In some cases, you may find a birth class that can educate you on both your primary and secondary delivery method (best possible and worst possible outcome).

- **Schedule -** We live in a society where we are constantly bombarded by the demands of our job, academics, families, etc. Selecting the right birth class means that you must consider you and your partner's daily schedule and compare it with your birth class's schedule to prevent clashes. If you have a hectic schedule, then explain your schedule to your birth class coordinator, so she or he can be flexible in helping you and knowing how much time and what time of the day you can devote to the class. For instance, most class coordinators can do home visits in the morning, afternoon, or evening at your convenience. They can even structure payment plans, and discounts to assist you based on your finances. You also want to make sure that you select a birth class that's within the vicinity of your home, school, or job. If it's closer to home, it'll be easy to transport back and forth. If it's minutes away from your job or school, you can easily transport from work or school to class.

Creditability - test the creditability of the class that you'll be signing up for by checking the reviews of that institution or individual on Google or by asking for certification. You may also test their credibility by asking to view their portfolio and seek testimonials from their past or present students.

Get Baby Stuff

Start stocking up on your nursery by buying the basics or asking for them as gifts. Essential items include baby clothes, blankets, nappies, baby wipes, and bum cream. Necessary equipment includes a car seat, a bassinet or cot where your baby will sleep, and possibly a pram or stroller. If you don't have the finances to accumulate these stuff, then you may want to consider creating an online baby registry, throwing a baby shower. These are the two most common and easiest way for people to bring gifts as a means of celebrating the life of your baby. You may also seek out second-hand items in great condition at significantly reduced prices.

Chapter Nine

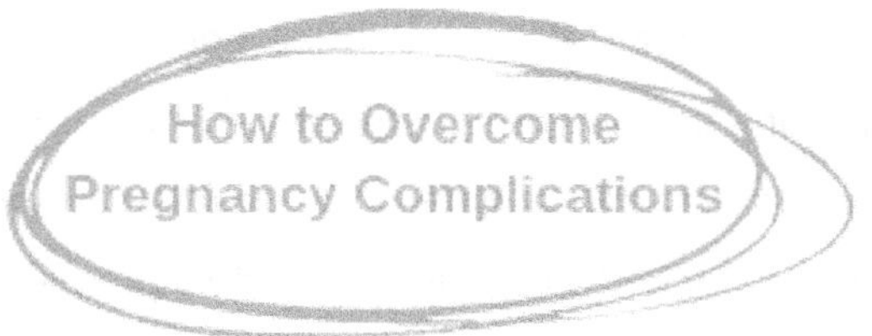

The American Diabetes Association states that gestational diabetes occurs when your body is not able to make and use all the insulin that's needed to break down glucose. Without enough insulin, glucose cannot leave the blood and be converted into energy. Glucose is then built up in the blood to high levels, which eventually results in gestational diabetes. Other research states that women with polycystic ovarian syndrome (PCOS) are also known to develop gestational diabetes later in their pregnancy even if they don't have a high sugar intake. This is as a result of their body's incapability to produce enough insulin to properly breakdown and digest the sugars from their meals. Studies have also shown that women with a high sugar diet can also develop gestational diabetes. Therefore, a well-balanced diet is recommended during pregnancy whether or not you have PCOS or high sugar intake.

How to Know if You Have Gestational Diabetes

Gestational diabetes typically develops between the 24th and 28th week of pregnancy. Therefore, most pregnant women will be advised by their health-care provider to have a glucose screening within that timeframe to determine if they have or do not have gestational diabetes. If you're near or beyond that time frame and your health-care provider hasn't mentioned anything about doing a glucose test, then I recommend that you talk to your health-care provider about it.

Some symptoms of gestational diabetes are fatigue, blurred vision, excessive thirst, excessive need to urinate, or snoring.

The Effects of Gestational Diabetes on Your Baby

Knowing how gestational diabetes can affect your baby can be a moment of enlightenment that motivates and keep you discipline about tackling the matter.

Here are a few effects of gestational diabetes on your baby:

- **Macrosomia -** Macrosomia is a medical term for excessive birth weight. This means that the size of your baby will be above the average because of the extra glucose in your bloodstream. Once excessive glucose is in your bloodstream, this will travel to your placenta, causing your baby to feed on it. Once your baby starts feeding on it, it causes your baby's pancreas to produce extra insulin and can cause your baby to grow beyond an average weight. A baby that's beyond the average weight can lead to a more difficult delivery. In some cases, an emergency c-section will be required.

- **Jaundice -** Jaundice is a common condition that is found in newborns whose mother has gestational diabetes. Jaundice is proven to take the form of a yellowish pigmentation of your baby's skin. It can also make the white areas of a baby's eyes appear yellow. This happens when there is too much bilirubin in their blood. This is nothing serious, and a special light is often used to get rid of the bilirubin pigment.

- **Learning Disability -** In recent studies, scientists have discovered that newborns are exposed to excessive sugar, whether from their mom having gestational diabetes or not. Babies are susceptible to faulty cognitive development, inconsistent mood behavior, non-verbal abilities, and impaired memory, among other future learning disabilities that will affect their baby until adolescence or adulthood. Whether you have gestational diabetes or not, you must maintain proper control of your sugar intake to give your child a fair chance of achieving a better life through cognitive intelligence.

The Effects of Gestational Diabetes on Mothers

Pregnant women who are diagnosed with gestational diabetes and don't manage it well are at a higher risk of having a cesarean section due to the large size of their baby. Observation also shows that women who don't manage their gestational diabetes well during their pregnancy are also at a higher risk of developing Type 2 diabetes after their pregnancy.

How to Treat Gestational Diabetes

While many medical practitioners may beat around the bush, we won't. The most effective way to treat gestational diabetes without taking medication is to simply manage what you eat. Your diet should include protein with the right inclusion of carbohydrates and fats.

Here's a list of the foods that you should eat:

- Fresh vegetables (uncooked or lightly steamed)

- Fresh fruits (You can still eat fruit if you have diabetes, however. you'll need to keep track of how much you're eating. You also need to strike a balance between eating sour and sweet fruits)

- Skinless chicken breasts

- Baked wild caught sea-fish

- Unsweetened Greek yogurt

- Whole-grain bread and oats

- Brown rice and pasta, quinoa or buckwheat, (Eat in small portions and according to how your body responds to it.)

- Whole-grain cereal

- Legumes, such as black beans, chickpeas, or kidney beans.

Eating from this food group means that you won't always stay full; therefore, you may want to increase your portion size or eat more small portions, according to how your body responds to it.

Tianka was unable to consume any vegetables during the first two trimesters of her pregnancy. The smell of cooked vegetables was a turn off for her. Whenever she consumed vegetables, she would regurgitate it. If this sounds familiar to you, then I understand your struggle. Not wanting to eat certain foods can be associated with a mental block. Therefore, you can cheat your way into eating vegetables by making vegetable smoothies along with a mixture of your favorite fruit to disguise the taste and smell of the vegetables.

A list of foods that you must avoid:

- Fast food

- Alcoholic beverages

- Baked goods, such as muffins, donuts, or cakes

- Fried food

- Sugary drinks, such as soda, juice, and sweetened beverages

- Candy (while you don't need to avoid sweets completely, you should monitor your intake closely as candy can raise your blood sugar quickly.)

- Very starchy foods, such as white potatoes and white rice

Insulin Management

Your health-care provider will recommend that you use a glucose monitor to test your blood sugar levels an hour after each meal. Doing a glucose test after each meal will help to let you know how that meal affected your sugar levels. By the food you ate and the results that you got from your glucose monitor, you'll be able to create a better meal plan that works for you.

Here's a list of glucose monitors that will provide accurate results:

- Contour Next EZ

- ReliON

- Abbott FreeStyle Lite

- Accu-Chek Aviva Connect

Tianka's choice of glucose monitor was - ReliOn. Above all, ensure that you are eating healthy.

How to Treat Carpal Tunnel Syndrome

Carpal tunnel syndrome can be treated as soon as its symptoms appear. Extreme measures such as surgery aren't necessary for carpal tunnel syndrome as it typically goes away within days, weeks, or months after your pregnancy. Some remedies for treating carpal tunnel syndrome include:

- **Massage-** Massage therapy is a perfect way to help relieve the discomfort, pain, tingling, or numbness that comes with carpal tunnel syndrome (CTS) as it will loosen and soothe tight muscles, and nerves.

- You don't need to break the bank for massage therapy. You can ask your partner or someone who you are comfortable with to gently massage your fingers, hands, wrist, shoulders, neck, and upper back.

- **Exercise** – Light exercises such as gently wiggling your fingers, making a fist, and then gently releasing your fist will help to release some pressure on the median nerve in your hand(s) and improve blood circulation.

- **Heat or Cold Therapy** – Cold therapy is known to provide pain and swelling relief for inflamed muscles, nerves, or joints. You can use this method by applying an ice pack, ice wrapped in a towel, or you can soak your wrist in cold water for 10 -15 minutes.

  Since the nerves (median nerve) that are being affected in your hand(s) are connected to your neck, shoulders, and upper back: you must also apply cold therapy to those areas to get the best results.

  Another alternative is hot therapy (Thermotherapy). Most experts believe that hot therapy is more effective than cold therapy because it is known to relax and loosen tight and inflamed nerves and muscles instantly. You can apply heat therapy by placing a heating pad, warm towel (soaked in warm water) to the inflamed area(s), and let it sit for 10-15 minutes. You can also soak your wrist in warm water at a bearable temperature. Since the nerves (median nerve) that are being affected in your hand(s) are connected to your neck, shoulders and upper back, you must also apply heat therapy to those areas to get the best results.

- **Rest** – Since bending and most other activities can cause further inflammation, it's highly recommended that you reduce intense activities that require you to use your hands. It's also important that you avoid sleeping on your hands.

Chapter Ten

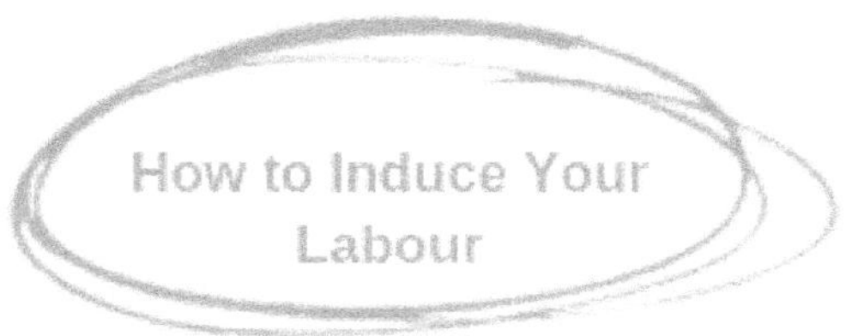

Due dates aren't always accurate. The word "due date" is also termed as "EDD," which means "Estimated Due Date." It's merely a calculated time of when your baby will potentially be 40 weeks and not when he or she will arrive. Therefore, don't be too alarmed by your worries, or by the worries of your health-care provider, family members, or friends when your baby hasn't arrived.

The reason why most babies are overdue is an unsolved puzzle. However, researchers say that your baby is more likely to be overdue if:

- This is your first pregnancy

- You've had a prior overdue pregnancy

- You're obese

- Hereditary

- Your due date was miscalculated due to confusion over the exact date of the start of your last menstrual period or if your due date was based on a late second or third-trimester ultrasound.

Medical Inducement Methods

In the first week of your due date, typically at 41 weeks, you and your baby are not yet at risk of complications. Therefore, there's no urgent need for the application of any of the medical inducement methods that I'm about to list. However, you are still in the safe zone, and you decide to utilize any medical inducement method based on convenience, instinct, your busy schedule, or because you simply want to get your baby out and get on with your life.

Once you've reached the 41 weeks mark, your health-care provider will administer various check-up such as ultrasound scans, as well as check your baby's movements and heartbeat to ensure that you and your baby are both healthy. They will also administer checks ups to determine whether it's better to use medical inducement methods or to keep the baby inside with close monitoring.

The common types of medical interventions that are offered to moms when they are overdue are:

- **Membrane sweep** – During a vaginal examination, your health-care provider will insert a finger into the opening of your cervix (neck of your womb) and then gently, but firmly move his or her finger around. This will separate the membranes of the amniotic sac surrounding your baby from your uterus. Once the membranes are ruptured, you will experience fluid leaking out of your vagina; This membrane separation releases hormones that are called prostaglandins. Prostaglandins can kick-start labor contractions in approximately 24-48 hours. Once a membrane sweep has been done, no other medical inducement method is usually required.

  In the case where a membrane sweep fails, most health-care providers will perform two or three membrane sweep before he or she suggests or performs other inducement methods.

  Risks: A membrane sweep procedure is quick, simple, and easy. However, a membrane sweep can be uncomfortable, as the cervix is difficult to reach before labor begins. Women who have their membrane swept multiple times are at risk of developing an infection, minor or excessive vaginal bleeding. Studies have shown that a membrane sweep is safe and carries minimal risk when it's performed by a certified professional.

- **Oxytocin-** According to the American Pregnancy Association, Pitocin and syntocinon are brand name medications that are forms of oxytocin. Oxytocin is a synthetic version of the natural oxytocin hormone that a pregnant woman's body produces. It works by stimulating your uterus, causing it to contract and trigger intense and consistent labor contractions. Once oxytocin is required, it will be applied intravenously into the vein.

Risks: Oxytocin is known to make contractions stronger, consistent, and more painful than the contractions that a woman experiences during natural labor. You are more likely to need pain relief, and your baby will continually be monitored.

Oxytocin is also known to speed up contractions, making the come too quickly. The speed of the contractions can affect your baby's heart rate by causing fetal distress. Once a baby is in fetal distress, an emergency cesarean surgery will be needed.

- **Artificial membrane rupture (breaking your water) –** An artificial membrane rupture is done when a woman's water doesn't break on its own. During a vaginal exam, your health-care provider will insert a long plastic device that looks like a big crochet needle, otherwise known as an amnihook, into your vagina and puncture a hole in the amniotic sac. Once the amniotic sac is punctured, you will experience water gushing from your vagina. Normally, your contractions will start coming stronger and faster once the amniotic sac is punctured. In some cases where an artificial membrane rupture has failed to start your contractions or has failed to maintain consistent and heavy contractions, you will be given oxytocin to get your contractions going and to maintain its strength and consistency.

Risks: Serious complications are rare with artificial membrane rupture. However, a few minor risks are that the baby may rotate in a breech position, making birth more complicated if the membranes are ruptured before head engagement. According to The National Center for Biotechnology Information-"The most common complication associated with an artificial rupture of membranes is a "prolapse of the umbilical cord." A prolapse of the umbilical cord occurs if an artificial rupture of membranes is performed when the baby's head is not fully engaged in the maternal pelvis.

In the case of an unengaged fetal head, the rupture of membranes may allow the umbilical cord to precede the fetal head when the release of amniotic fluid occurs. This will allow the fetal head to compress the section of umbilical cord preceding the head, generally leading to fetal bradycardia and a possible emergency cesarean section. There is an increased risk of infection if there is a prolonged time between rupture and birth.

- **Prostaglandin** – This is a synthetic version of the natural prostaglandin hormone that's created by a pregnant woman's body to kick start labor. Prostaglandin hormone is inserted during a vaginal examination as a gel, pessary, and tape (similar to a tampon) or as a tablet. It is typically done overnight in the hospital to make the cervix "ripe." The cervix will soften, shorten, and opens. The uterus then starts to contract regularly for delivery.

Risks: Studies have shown that vaginal prostaglandins increase the likelihood of vaginal birth within 24 hours. However, they can also over-stimulate the uterus, causing it to contract too much and slow down the baby's heart rate. Some women find that their vagina is too sore after the prostaglandin procedure, or they might experience nausea, vomiting, or diarrhea.

Natural Inducement Methods

If you prefer not to use any of the above medical inducing methods, here are a few natural inducing methods that are used globally by midwives and most medical practitioners.

- **Sexual Penetration** – You don't need a prescription for it. Therefore, have a lot of sex! Sex during pregnancy, as well as before or after your due date, is safe, extremely potent, and beneficial. Research shows that a lot of women have had success with inducing labor just by having sex. Sexual penetration is known to stimulate the cervix, causing it to release Prostaglandin. Sperms are also known to contain prostaglandins. Therefore, when sperms are released inside of the cervix, it may act as a natural source of prostaglandins for cervical ripening that can help with dilation. Also, a woman's orgasm during intercourse may lead to cervix ripening, causing the uterus to cramp or to contract. It may be more sex than you want to have, but it certainly beats the medical alternative.; all of which come with high-risk factors.

- **Nipple stimulation** – Nipple stimulation is known to trigger the pituitary gland to release oxytocin, which brings on cramping and contractions. Nipple stimulation can be done by yourself, your partner, or with a breast pump. A slow rhythmic massage of the breast behind the areola (the ring of darker skin surrounding the nipple) between your fingers is the best technique for inducing your labor. Once your health-care provider approves that you are fit for this method, you can manually stimulate your nipples. Your partner can stimulate your nipples orally; if you have an older baby whom you're still nursing, you can use him or her to stimulate your nipples through breastfeeding.

- **Massage therapy/Acupressure –** Massage therapy as an inducing method produces chemicals in the body that initiate contractions. Getting frequent massages from your partner or a masseuse can help prepare you mentally and physically. Acupressure is also a great traditional Chinese practice that targets specific areas of your body that are believed to raise your body's level of oxytocin and bring on labor contractions. A professional masseuse will focus on these specific pressure points.

- **Walking –** When it comes to inducing labor, walking is the safest and simplest inducing method there is, yet, it's overlooked. Research shows that during walking, the rhythmic pressure of your baby's head on your cervix stimulates the release of oxytocin. Oxytocin is that hormone you'll need to help spur and regulate your contractions. It's important not to wear yourself out; therefore, you should go for short and slow walks.

- **Essentials oils** - When it comes to inducing labor, essential oils are a great option because they are very potent. Essential oils are "highly concentrated aromatic extracts that are distilled from a variety of plants, leaves, and flowers. Among the many types of essentials oils that are on the market; here are a few that have been used for inducing labor by midwives for decades:

- **Clary Sage Oil -** This therapeutic plant oil is known to allow the muscles to release tension and relax, thus naturally encouraging contractions.

- **Evening Primrose Oil –** This essential oil is commonly known as a healing oil. It's categorized as a cervical ripening agent because it can have a significant impact on fastening the progression of labor by softening the cervix, which is usually the first step in labor induction. It's known to have side effects such as: thinning out the blood, nausea, headaches, or stomachache during the process. Therefore, it is best to use evening primrose oil along with other essential oil blends so that the other essential oils can counter the side effects of evening primrose oil.

Jasmine Oil: Jasmine oil is known for its sweet alluring smell. It can be used during labor as it offers pain relief during each stage of labor. It's also known to hasten labor by intensifying contractions and ensuring the smooth advancement of labor.

How to apply essential oils: Essential oils can be applied topically to your pressure points such as the inner ankle, abdomen area, hips, pelvis, lower back, or as indicated by your health-care provider. You may also inhale it to start the inducing process.

There are a lot more essential oils that are beneficial for inducing labor. However, the three essential oils that are listed above are oils that Tianka utilized. If you're curious about using or learning about other essential oils that are beneficial for labor inducement, then I recommend that you first consult with your health-care provider. Essential oils are extremely potent, and unless you are ready to have your baby, then do not use it. Once you have decided that you're going to use essential oils as a part of your pregnancy or labor, please speak to your health-care provider before using any essential oils during pregnancy or labor.

- **Pineapple Juice** – Pineapple contains a type of enzyme called proteolytic bromelain that helps to induce labor by softening the cervix. Eating pineapple in large amounts also stimulates your stomach, which then causes contractions in your uterus and kick-starts labor.

- **Red raspberry leaf tea** –Red raspberry leaf tea is known to strengthen the uterus and pelvic wall when consumed during pregnancy. Because of its stimulating effects, most midwives don't recommend drinking until your second trimester. For inducing labor, you'll want to increase your dosage of this tea to help kick-start labor.

Every woman's body and pregnancy will respond differently to inducing methods. Therefore, no method(s) is guaranteed to introduce you to labor. Also, both medical or natural induction methods are reserved for pregnant women who are 39 weeks pregnant or over and whose body and baby are at a level of optimal health to undergo medical or natural inducing methods. Therefore, it's imperative that you first consult your health-care provider who's been following your nine-months journey before attempting any inducing method.

Chapter Eleven

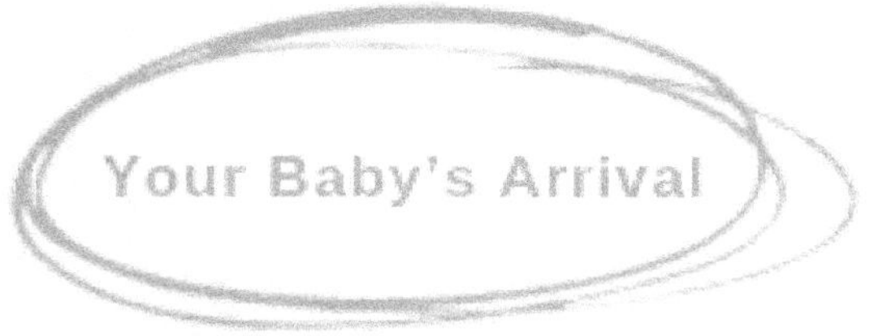

God's promise to you is that He'll never leave or forsake you and that He's with you wherever you go. Therefore, it doesn't matter where (home or hospital) or how (natural childbirth, medicated childbirth, or cesarean section) your baby was born. If you and your baby made it safely outside of the walls of the hospital, then you experienced a supernatural birth. Whatever your outcome is, always remember that you should never compare your birth story to that of others. Your birth story is unique, and to compare it to other people's birth story means that you haven't comprehended just how graceful and blessed you are. Therefore, rejoice!

Resources

Sample Birth Plan

Mother's Name:

____

Mother's Date of Birth:

____

Father's Name:

____

Father's Date of Birth:

____

Expected Due Date:

____

Type of Delivery:

____

Birth Location & Address:

____

____

____

Primary Health-Care Provider's Name:

____

____

Secondary Health-Care Provider's Name:

____

____

Secondary Health-Care Provider's Address:

____

____

____

<h2 style="text-align:center">In Early Labor I plan on:</h2>

This section should contain all the things you want to do during the early stages of labor. For example:

- Eat and drink light food.

- Take short walks and light stretches.

- Resting.

- Take hot or cold showers.

- Do light activities to keep my mind off the clock.

- Make phone calls to update family members and friends.

- Be alone with my partner as much as possible

<h2 style="text-align:center">In Active Labor I plan on:</h2>

This section should contain all the things you want to do during active labor. For example:

- To be asked whenever a cervical check may be required.

- Intermittent fetal monitoring with a Doppler.

- Intermittent fetal monitoring with a fetoscope.

- To be left to myself and my partner while coping as much as possible.

- Minimal touching or talking while I'm in labor except for my partner.

My Birth Support Team

This section should contain all the people who are apart of your birth support team and their roles. For example:

I would like to have my birth team surround me and help me as outlined:

- **(Partner/Father)** – He will provide affirmations, spiritual declarations, physical touch, and comfort. He will also help me cope through labor and be my main source of support for guiding exercises, birthing, and relaxation with suggestions from the midwife only when necessary.

- **Aunt** - She will provide moral support and help with keeping supplies ready for hot and cool compresses. She also will help to provide light meals and drink throughout labor as needed or requested.

- **Sister** – She will help with filming the moment and capturing pictures. She will also ensure that family members who are not physically present can tune in and be a part of the birth via Skype and other video calling methods.

- **Cousin** – She will also help with filming the moment and capturing pictures. She will also ensure that family members who are not present can tune in and be a part of the birth via Skype and other video calling methods. She should also be allowed to observe all aspects of the birth process, from a medical student's perspective so she can hopefully advocate for a natural birth or be a witness to a true natural uninterrupted birth.

Pain Relief Methods

This section should contain your preferred pain relief substance or method (Natural or medicated) that you'll be using to manage your pain during labor and delivery.

For example:

- I want hot compresses or cool cloth for areas on my body that ache, along with breathing techniques.

- To be reminded to make low deep sounds.

- To be reminded to relax and breathe the baby down.

- To be reminded to change positions (hands and knees, squatting, standing, sitting on the birth ball, left side lying, sitting on the toilet).

- I want to take a warm shower.

- To labor in the birth pool.

- A specific playlist to be on when requested.

- I want to be massaged by my partner or family member when requested.

- I want essential oils to be diffused in the air.

In Birth (Pushing) I plan on:

This section should contain all the things you want to do during childbirth. For example:

- Deliver in water (Birth tub).

- To push instinctively, in my own way, in my own time as long as the baby and I are not at risk

- To be reminded to make low deep sounds

- To be reminded to relax and breathe the baby out.

- To be reminded to change positions (hands and knees, squatting, standing, classic, etc.

- To be offered a mirror to see the baby crowning.

- I want my midwife to count when I push.

- To have photos taken of the pushing stage.

- To have my partner catch the baby.

- To remain in the water until the placenta is delivered.

- To leave the cord attached until it stops pulsating (and even longer for pictures.)

- I want my partner to cut the cord.

- I want myself or my partner to be present while all the newborn exams and procedures are being done.

- No mother-baby separation

Newborn Decisions

This section should contain all the things that you do not want to be administered to your child after birth. For example:

I have discussed and know the risks and benefits of the following newborn informed choices, and I would prefer:

- Do not administer Erythromycin Eye Prophylaxis.

- Do not administer Vitamin K drops orally or injectable.

- Do not apply the Pulse Ox to my baby during the newborn exam.

- Please do not perform the newborn metabolic screen.

In Case of Hospital Transfer, I would Prefer:

This section should contain all the things you want to be administered in case of a hospital transfer. For example:

- To keep my birth support team with me.

- Please do not offer pain medication unless I ask for it.

- To avoid pain medication in case of vaginal delivery.

- I agree to an IV of fluids.

- To allow the cord to stop pulsating before father cuts it.

- To place baby skin to skin as soon as possible after birth.

In Case of a Cesarean Birth, I would Prefer:

This section should contain all the things you want to be administered in case of a cesarean section. For example:

- To be awake.

- To have my partner with me during birth (I understand if general anesthesia is needed, my partner is unable to be with me).

- To place baby skin to skin as soon as possible after birth.

- To allow the cord to stop pulsating before the father cuts it.

- I want my partner to be present while all the newborn exams and procedures are being done.

- That someone from my birth support team is with me in the recovery room.

Postpartum Newborn Decisions I would Prefer:

- My partner and I to be informed of all procedures that will be performed on my newborn.

- To keep my baby with me until he or she has breastfed successfully on both sides.

- To exclusively breastfeed, please no artificial nipples, formula or sugar water.

- Do not administer Erythromycin Eye Prophylaxis.

- Administer Vitamin K drops orally.

- Please do not perform the Newborn Metabolic Screen.

- Do not administer the Hep B Vaccine.

Your Birth Plan

This section is for you to customize your birth plan based on your preferences with the help of the sample birth plan above.

Mother's Name: _______________________________

Mother's Date of Birth: _______________________________

Father's Name: _______________________________

Father's Date of Birth: _______________________________

Expected Due Date: _______________________________

Type of Delivery : _______________________________

Birth Location & Address:

____

____

____

____

____

Primary Health-Care Provider's Name:

____

____

____

Secondary Health-Care Provider's Name:

____

____

____

Secondary Health-Care Provider's Location:

____

____

____

____

____

____

In Early Labor I plan on:

____

____

____

____

____

____

____

In Active Labor I plan on:

My Birth Support Team:

Pain Relief:

In Birth (Pushing) I plan on:

Newborn Decisions:

In Case of Hospital Transfer, I Prefer:

In Case of a Cesarean Birth, I Prefer:

____

____

____

____

____

____

____

____

____

____

____

____

Postpartum Newborn Decisions I Prefer:

About the Author

Georgandez is the husband of Tianka Morrison and founder of virtu. After the birth of his first child, Geor'nyah Morrison, Georgandez didn't want strangers to raise his daughter. Then he founded Virtual Media Hive, an online company that provides services such as virtual assistance, website design, Logo design, social media management, content creation, videography, and photography to public figures, startups, and established companies.

Learn more by visiting: virtualmediahive.com

His lifetime goals are to father a healthy and functional family, to fulfill his God-given destiny, and to keep sharing life's most important lessons through his unusual style of writing the end of a book before the beginning. Outside of his passion for writing, he can be caught red-handed making an iced cold mango passion fruit smoothie after a long morning walk.

Georgandez has a genuine love for people, therefore, connect with Georgandez on his social platforms:

Georgandez Morrison

Facebook: Georgandez Morrison

Instagram: @georgandez

Youtube: The Morrisons Tv

Email: georgandezmorrison@gmail.com

Tianka Morrison

Facebook: Tianka Morrison

Instagram: @tiankamorrison

Youtube: The Morrisons Tv